SO YOU WANT TO BE A DOULA

The Indispensable Guide to Match You to Your Perfect Doula Career

CARRIE KENNER

Copyright © 2024 Carrie Kenner

All rights reserved.

No part of this publication may be reproduced, distributed, or transmitted in any form or by any means, including photocopying, recording, or other electronic or mechanical methods, without the prior written permission of the publisher, except as permitted by U.S. copyright law. For permission requests, contact the author at: carrie@carriekenner.com.

ISBN Paperback: 979-8-9918071-0-4
ISBN eBook: 979-8-9918071-1-1

Publisher's Cataloging-in-Publication Data

Names: Kenner, Carrie, author.

Title: So you want to be a doula : the indispensable guide to match you to your perfect doula career / Carrie Kenner.

Description: Olympia, WA: SunWaterTrees Press, 2024.

Identifiers: LCCN: 2024922177 | ISBN: 979-8-9918071-0-4 (paperback) | 979-8-9918071-1-1 (ebook)

Subjects: LCSH Doulas. | Caregivers. | BISAC BUSINESS & ECONOMICS / Careers / General

Classification: RG950 .K46 2024 | DDC 618.4--dc23

This publication is designed to provide accurate and authoritative information for people interested in becoming a doula. The content provided herein is for educational purposes only and does not take the place of formal doula training, or business, tax, or legal advice from an attorney. Every effort has been made to ensure that the content provided is accurate and helpful for readers at the time of publishing. However, this is not an exhaustive treatment of the subject.

No liability is assumed for losses or damages due to the information provided. You are responsible for your own choices, actions, and results. While the publisher and author have used their best efforts in preparing this book, they make no representations or warranties with respect to the accuracy or completeness of the contents of this book and specifically disclaim any implied warranties. The advice and strategies contained herein may not be suitable for your situation. Neither the publisher nor the author shall be liable for any loss of profit or any other commercial damages, including but not limited to special, incidental, consequential, personal, or other damages.

Cover design and Illustration: Andrea Gabriel
Interior design: Ayeshan

Published by SunWaterTrees Press

Printed in the U.S.A.

For information about special discounts available for bulk purchases, sales promotions, or educational needs, contact the author at carrie@carriekenner.com.

First edition 2024 ⁕ Printed in the United States of America

Well, this wasn't the one you were waiting to see, Mom, but it's the one I got done first. I'm sorry you aren't here to hold it in your hands. But I know you're just as proud.

"Don't ask what the world needs. Ask what makes you come alive, and go do it. Because what the world needs is people who have come alive."

—Howard Thurman, civil rights activist

"Our prime purpose in this life is to help others. And if you can't help them, at least don't hurt them."

—Dalai Lama, spiritual leader, peace activist

Contents

Part 1 : You Are Here

Introduction 3

Chapter 1 - Your Future as a Doula..9

Chapter 2 - Who This Book Is For 17

Chapter 3 - What Is a Doula?..23

Chapter 4 - The History and Breadth of the Doula Movement.................31

Chapter 5 - What's Stopping You? 39

Part 2 : The Become a Doula Framework

Chapter 6 - Step 1: What Kind of Doula Role Are You
    Interested In?..47

Chapter 7 - Step 2: Your Lifestyle Assessment 67

Chapter 8 - Step 3: Doula Role Variables 77

Chapter 9 - Step 4: The Doula-bility Calculator 91

Chapter 10 - What Does It Take to Be a Doula?..103

Part 3 : Find the Training That's Right for You

Chapter 11 - Your Learning Style(s) 119

Chapter 12 - Know Your Training Options..127

Chapter 13 - Researching Doula Trainings 139

Chapter 14 - Your Top Three Training Options 147

Chapter 15 - How to Fund Your Doula Training..................................155

Chapter 16 - Alternatives to Formal Doula Training 159

Part 4 : Preparing for a Doula Career

Chapter 17 - Is There a Demand for Doulas?...................................167

Chapter 18 - Marketing and Finding Clients 171

Chapter 19 - Business Basics...185

Chapter 20 - Community and Family Support 201

Chapter 21 - Ongoing Coaching and Doula Communities 205

Closing - Is the Doula Lifestyle for You? 207

Acknowledgments 209

About the Author..211

More From the Author 215

So you want to be a doula. How does that feel in this moment…

hearing the call…

to something that totally stirs your heart?

At the most basic level, being a doula means making the world a better place for *others*.

Doulas want to be of service to people, helping them go through something difficult (often something they themselves have gone through) or something they recognize as challenging for most people.

They want to make life a bit easier and kinder.

Doulas also tend to be rabble-rousers.

They have a passion for helping the underdog. They see the world a bit outside of the box.

Doulas want to create change.

They aren't ass-kissers or "yes" people. They want to affect social change through heart-centered services versus blowing shit up or moving at the glacier-like speed of legislation.

Whatever brought you here, whatever version of doula you desire to be, I am so glad you are here.

Welcome!

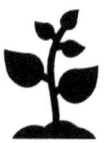

Part 1

You Are Here

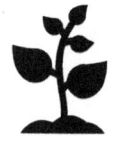

INTRODUCTION

If you opened this book, you must have some interest in doulas. Maybe you recently heard the word *doula*, and are just learning what a doula does. Or maybe you've been researching doulas for months or years and are ready to finally become one.

Wherever you are in your personal journey, I'm glad my book gets to be a part of it.

This book exists for four reasons:

1. To help you fulfill your dream of becoming a doula
2. To help you figure out the best doula role for your current lifestyle
3. To prevent you from wasting time and money on the wrong doula training
4. To introduce you to me and my body of work, in the hope that I can continue to support your journey

How am I going to do all that?

With my *Become a Doula* framework. There are three parts to my unique framework for preparing doulas:

1. Determine which doula role is a good fit for you and your current lifestyle
2. Find a doula training that matches your learning style and that you will complete
3. Prepare you to get your doula career off to a good start so you are ready to get clients and create a successful business

Part 1: Figure out what kind of doula role is best suited for you.

I'm going to tell you all the things you need to know about various doula roles. Being a doula is a combination of interests, skills, and feasibility. For example, you may be fascinated by birth but have young children at home. Can you be on call and leave your kids at a moment's notice to go to a birth? If you want to help people navigate the court system, are you available to support them during their court session if you have a day job?

Many people want to be a doula based on their area of interest, passion, or experience (birth, postpartum, death, divorce, medical, etc.). But they may not understand the requirements for that doula role. You need to know where you'll be doing most of your work, what the hours might be, how flexible the work is (or isn't), who you'll be working with primarily, or what the work entails physically, emotionally, mentally, or spiritually.

You're going to learn about twenty-six different doula roles to find the best match for you. A series of assessment tools will help you determine which roles will be a good fit for your personality, interests, lifestyle, and needs. Finally, the *Doula-bililty Calculator* will help you put it all together and find the doula roles you are most likely to succeed at now.

Once you've figured out what doula role will work for you, you have to get trained, and there may be many training options to choose from.

Part 2: Find the best training for you.

I'll show you how to determine your learning styles, understand the features of various trainings, and how to research them to compare features and assess a good fit for you. I'm going to warn you what to watch out for in a training. And I'm going to tell you about my trainings and why I structure them the way I do, to see if that helps you understand what to look for in a training.

You'll use my *Find-a-Training Tool* to identify your top three training options and select the one you will use.

Also, some doula fields don't have formal training, so I'll show you alternative ways to equip yourself with doula skills and knowledge in your field.

Once you are trained, it's time to start doula-ing!

Part 3: Start getting clients and launch your career.

The final piece of my framework is showing you how to start and build your doula career after you've taken your training. You'll learn about different business structures, what to expect when starting a business, and how to find clients to ensure you are ready to go when your training is complete.

I'll share the main strategies and steps in Chapter 18. You'll know what you have to do to be a successful doula *while you are learning to become one.* **This is the best defense against *learning* how to be a doula but not *doing* it!**

You'll also learn about systems you can put in place to create a sustainable business, such as lifestyle, self-care, and finances. I'll show you the steps to attract your ideal clients, market your services, and create meaningful relationships that serve both you and your clients.

❋ ❋ ❋

There are many ways to become a doula. I think mine is the best approach for many people, but not for everyone. This book will help you figure out if my process and style is a good fit for you.

If it is, follow my steps and you will become successful in your new career.

After you complete this book, you'll take your chosen training and then put all the components together.

My goal is for you to start building your doula business before you've completed your training, so you are set up for success. Then I invite you to join my cohort of doulas to fully launch and grow your business in the first year.

Being a doula is relational work, and doulas need other people who understand the job to bounce ideas off, to debrief and process tough situations with, and to inspire them to keep going. You'll learn about the benefits of ongoing coaching, doula communities, and my doula business coaching program to ensure your success.

Here's the magic of my approach, summed up in these three points:

> **Point #1:** Too many times, people want to be a doula without knowing what it entails. This book will give you a realistic understanding of multiple doula roles to find the one you can succeed in.
>
> **Point #2:** People spend thousands of dollars on doula trainings that don't provide what they need in a format they can digest. I'll show you how to assess and choose a training that you'll actually learn from and complete.
>
> **Point #3:** For decades, doulas have struggled to create a successful career because they didn't know they'd have to start a business or they didn't know how to. I wrote Part 4: Preparing for a Doula Career in this book to change all that.

While this is a book about how to become a doula, it's also a book about how to follow your dreams and make the world a better place. You will be transformed as you embody the essence of being a doula, develop skills you never dreamed of, discover job freedom, and serve your community in a heart-centered way.

Ultimately, I want the world to be filled with doulas for all of life's challenging situations, and I want *you* to be one of those doulas. I believe doulas DO change the world, one birth, baby, death, divorce, [fill in the blank] at a time.

After you read this book, if you need help choosing or launching your doula career, please visit my website at www.doula-training.carriekenner.com to sign up for a course or schedule a chat.

I've created this training program to get you started: **Become a Doula:** *Foundational Training for All Types of Doulas.*

Introduction

If your dream is to become a birth doula and that role is a good fit for you, I hope you'll consider my *Becoming a Birth Doula* online training (that is, if online training is also a good fit for you).

Once you've completed your doula training, if you'd like to launch your business under my guidance and with the support of an entire community, I invite you to join my *JumpStart Your Doula Career* business coaching program.

It's my honor to share what I've learned in the past twenty-plus years as a birth doula and trainer to thousands of doulas. I'll intersperse bits of advice and lessons I've learned from my personal experiences, and from my doula colleagues in a multitude of doula roles.

Helping you become a doula and coaching your business to a place that brings you joy, financial reward, and pride is my zone of genius. I'm here to help.

To your success!

Carrie

❋ ❋ ❋

Many people consider the process of becoming a doula a journey. A personal journey, a soul journey, a spiritual journey. I certainly do.

If that idea resonates with you, I encourage you to get a copy of the *Becoming a Doula Journal* to track your process of becoming a doula. It's a gorgeous book where you can write, draw, and process your experience in a mindful and heartfelt way.

CHAPTER 1

Your Future as a Doula

It was 2001. I'd just turned forty. I had a newborn baby. My father had died two months ago—while I was eight months pregnant—and a few weeks after that, I got laid off from the company I'd been with for sixteen years.

You often hear people say, "Out of adversity comes opportunity." I sure as hell hoped so!

This confluence of events opened a doorway that I'd been wanting to step through for many years, which was starting my own business. I didn't know what kind of business it was going to be. I thought maybe I'd be a race director or an event organizer or a wedding planner.

But instead—because I was in the midst of pregnancy, birth, and postpartum and had just heard the word *doula* for the first time—*birth doula* is what grabbed my attention.

At that time, only three organizations trained birth doulas in North America. Everything, of course, was in person. Lucky for me, I lived in Seattle, Washington, where a birth doula training was held regularly. I took it and started doing the things to start my new business.

At the time, there was a nascent internet: no Wix, no Squarespace, no online courses. For bootstrap entrepreneurs on the brink of the technology boom, it was bleak. You had to DIY it or die. If you didn't have that start-from-scratch ability, you had to have money to pay someone to start it for you.

I didn't have money, but I had an old-school work ethic and dug in. I took free classes from the Small Business Administration, wrote and printed brochures on my home printer, and learned how to create a website with an instruction manual.

I was fortunate to live in a place where doulas were more well-known than other parts of the country, and where the community of doulas was very supportive of each other. In my first year, I attended fifteen births. In subsequent years I attended twenty-five to forty.

I followed the different directions my path was taking me: childbirth education, postpartum doula, lactation specialist. After three years, I was invited to be a doula trainer. I found mentors for each step of my journey: colleagues who were a few steps ahead of me, business coaches, and marketing experts.

I worked as a full-time birth doula for fifteen years. Through a process of understanding human psychology, presence, and trial and error, I discovered a way to get hired more often and easily have a full schedule as a doula.

I continually expanded my expertise and offerings. I retired from doula-ing in 2015 to focus full-time on training doulas. By 2018, I had trained over two thousand birth doulas, created eight advanced doula trainings, and hosted annual retreats and conferences for birth professionals. I've coached and mentored hundreds of doulas as they launched their doula businesses. And now, I'm a business and marketing coach for doulas and other small business owners.

I've proven that one can make a good living as a full-time doula and expand their work by creating courses, additional products, or specialty services.

And for yourself, you only have to look at the rise of doulas in the media and a plethora of doula trainings to realize doulas are hot!

Today, there are over one hundred *birth* doula training organizations or businesses, sixty postpartum doula trainings, twenty for death doulas, and hundreds of miscellaneous doula training companies.

There are no reliable ways to calculate the number of practicing doulas (or how many clients they serve or how much money they make), but we know that doulas are in the headlines of major newspapers and magazines almost daily.

"Maternity care in rural areas is in crisis. Can more doulas help?" — NPR, Jul 26, 2024

"The trend of Black women using doulas to overcome maternal death rates" — CBS News, Feb 22, 2024

"Massachusetts expands use of doula services to cut rates of infant mortality" — Boston 25 News, Apr 9, 2024

"Doula Care Has Gone Virtual" — The New York Times, Jun 10, 2024

"Hiring a Doula: Everything to Know, According to Expert" — Elle magazine, May 22, 2024

And the statistics on the benefits of doulas are unquestionable.

A Story of Doula Research

Quite a bit of research has been done on the impact of birth doulas. That research has shown conclusively that the presence of a doula lowers the rate of cesareans and premature births, and shortens the length of labor[1]; reduces the incidence of inductions, use of pain medications, and postpartum adjustment disorders[2]; and increases satisfaction with one's birth experience[3], regardless of how the birth unfolds.

What makes the data especially compelling is that research done in the early 1980s in birth facilities in Guatemala showed that **the simple presence of another person in the birthing room, without providing any direct support to the person in labor**, shortened the length of labor and decreased the amount of pain medications used[4]. These studies simply had a woman sit in the corner of the room knitting, or behind a curtain in the room, proving the point that **people do not want to be alone in labor** (author's note: or other emotionally-charged life situations).

Later research done in the 1990s showed that labor support provided by a trained person who was not a clinical provider and not a friend or relative of the birthing person (in other words, a doula) had better outcomes than labor support provided by 1) a clinical provider trained in labor support, or 2) a friend or relative trained in labor support. Both 1) and 2) improved outcomes—but not to the extent that a doula did[5].

You might wonder why the familiar friend or relative didn't have more of a positive impact than a stranger. Even though trained in what to expect and how to support birth, loved ones lack the objectivity that a doula brings. While friends and family members can provide calm, comfort, and information, they can be biased and influential, so it is best to pick your known ones wisely.

That same research also showed that the most significant benefits from doulas occurred in hospitals that normally didn't allow any support people, had the highest rates of interventions, and had the worst birth outcomes overall. Wherever people are least supported, doulas provide the most benefit[6].

What all of this research tells us is this: having someone familiar to a person in labor, and dedicated to providing emotional support and encouragement, makes a big difference in how the birth process works and how people feel about themselves and their experience after the birth.

1. https://pmc.ncbi.nlm.nih.gov/articles/PMC10292163/
2. https://pubmed.ncbi.nlm.nih.gov/7402234/
3. Listening to Mothers II Report
4. https://pubmed.ncbi.nlm.nih.gov/2013951/
5. Childbirth Connection. "Best Evidence: Labor Support." 2011.
6. Childbirth Connection. "Best Evidence: Labor Support." 2011.

What can we learn from this research that applies to all doulas?

1. People do not want to be alone during challenging life situations.
2. People don't need a lot of "stuff" done to them; they mainly need continuous attention from someone they already know and trust.
3. Technical care is not what makes people feel well-supported.
4. The support that people receive has to be objective, non-judgmental, and compassionate.
5. The systems with the least support built in lead to the worst outcomes and will benefit the most from doula support.

Being an Advocate *and* an Activist

You may think that you are coming into doula work to be an advocate for a certain type of outcome, such as winning a divorce case, finally getting pregnant, beating cancer, or having a natural birth. You might think that clients will want you to tell them what to do, or make decisions based on the information you provide after you educate them. But that is not how being a doula works.

A bit of information *might* be the key that unlocks a door to a different way of thinking. Your opinions *might* be asked for (and heeded). Your support *might* help someone speak up for themself. Or they might not.

Think of your role as an impartial mentor with the goal of helping your clients discover what *they* want and asking for your guidance to get there, all while supporting them along the way, especially if what they want isn't possible.

As a modern doula, you will be called upon to be an emissary for your chosen field in your community and in society. There are still many people around the world who have never heard the word, or have misunderstandings of what a doula is or does. For example, birth doulas are often depicted as crystal-toting hippies or bossy natural-birth evangelists on TV or in movies. You may have to do a lot of educating to change stereotypes.

As a doula, you will have to describe what a doula does over and over and over. You will repeatedly have to explain the difference between doulas and midwives, coaches, mediators, counselors, etc. You will have to educate people that doulas work with clinicians and professionals, people giving birth or dying, people too scared or nervous to advocate for themselves, and people who are all too often unheard and marginalized.

You may find yourself advocating for human rights or lobbying for legislative changes. Doulas have fought for the rights of people to choose who they want to accompany them in courtrooms, hospital rooms, and abortion clinics. They have lobbied to legalize midwifery in their state, for the right to nurse their children in public, for the right to refuse or withhold consent of treatments, for doula care to be covered by health insurance and Medicaid, and many other human rights issues.

The number of people who can be helped by the presence of a doula is endless. Thank you, doulas!

Now It's Your Turn

Congratulations on wanting to become a doula! It is one of the most rewarding jobs in the world. But it's more than a job… it's an identity, a calling, an act of service. It's also an entirely unique role because so few people actually know what a doula is, much less what they do.

There is a lot you will discover as you become a doula, not only about the doula role, but also about yourself, your future work as a doula, and the impact doulas have on big issues like mental health, mortality, humanity, and justice. There are many things to consider, but don't get bogged down by all the details yet, because the whole purpose of this book is to prepare you with information, tools, and skills to navigate the challenges of becoming and serving as a doula.

The first tool to help you become a great doula is something you already possess: *your desire*.

Your Desire to Become a Doula

What drives you to become a doula? It could be a belief that all medical patients should be respected and feel empowered, or a desire to make birth safer or more respectful for marginalized people. Some doulas have a goal to protect the financial status of people going through divorce, or to provide dignity to the dying. Nearly all people who are called to this line of work start with an interest or passion for a specific challenging time in life.

At first, your vision may include working with clients one-on-one. You can make a tremendous impact one person or family at a time. Over time, you may find your passion growing into activism, running a community-based organization, or expanding your services to make larger-scale impacts on communities and culture.

Being a doula is about having infinite compassion, highly-developed communication skills, the ability to be a source of strength in any situation, and a mysterious attraction to life situations that most people shy away from.

Whatever desire or passion drew you here, I know it will evolve and deepen as you continue to read. There may be some revelations along the way. You might not end up working in an area you expected, or you could end up being the busiest doula in your field. You might be a doula for decades, or switch gears in a year or two to try a new role or find a completely different arena to work in.

If you want to explore how your identity will change as you become a doula, get my companion guide, *Becoming a Doula Journal*, to help track your inner terrain.

How can following the call to become a doula change the world, and transform you in the process?

That is the question you will explore as I guide you through the process of transformation, not only in becoming a doula, but in discovering a deeper sense of self. No matter your path, I can guarantee one thing: you will be transformed by learning about the role of the doula.

As you step into this world, you can track your development by journaling your thoughts and ideas as they come up. Throughout the journal, there are activities, assignments, and prompts all designed to guide you in your evolution as a doula.

I also host an online support community for anyone on the road to becoming a doula. Visit www.doula-training.carriekenner.com/resources to join me there.

CHAPTER 2

Who This Book Is For

This book is the result of my life's greatest purpose: to support people who are oppressed or marginalized. How that manifested for me primarily was as a birth doula. I supported people in one of the most fraught, physically and emotionally challenging, spiritually profound, historically oppressed, and systemically disrespected experiences of life. Because birth is also racialized and medical care is a social justice issue, it garnered all my attention.

But there are many kinds of doulas. Birth and postpartum doulas, death or end-of-life doulas, divorce or court doulas, surgery or medical doulas. Which one is your calling? Which one is right for you?

This book is for you if:

▶ you are thinking about becoming a doula.

▶ you're already a doula (or in the helping professions) and want to expand your role.

▶ you want to help people through emotionally and/or physically challenging situations one-on-one—not as a clinical or technical expert but as a knowledgeable and caring guide.

Birth and pregnancy were my intellectual playground. The birth space was my comfort zone. Babies were my muse. Marginalized people are my heart. Helping people is my soul.

I tried being a postpartum doula and it didn't excite me, but lactation was a place I excelled. As my children grew older and my reproductive days faded, my attention to pregnancy and birth waned and my interest in death appeared (also fed by infant deaths and the courageous parents I'd witnessed).

My reputation as a listener, advocate, and someone who could navigate unfamiliar systems spread, and soon I was asked to support people on their journey with a brain tumor diagnosis, a miscarriage, a pregnancy termination, and knee surgery.

When my son was arrested and our family was catapulted into the court and prison system, we all would have benefited from someone who had walked this path before us. During my divorce, I wished I had a doula by my side—and later found out divorce doulas do exist.

All doulas come to this work as a result of their personal experiences or innate interests, or after hearing the word doula. And just as doulas want to support others through their experiences, I want to support you in the process of becoming one.

What I'm going to show you in this book is how to become the right kind of doula for you, where to learn how to be a doula, and how to get clients so you have a career that flourishes. Because without clients, you're not doula-ing.

If you want to learn about many different doula roles—not just the one you think you want to do—and learn about who your ideal clients will be, keep reading.

If you want to find a doula training that will provide you with the information and skills for your vision, don't put this book down.

If you want guidance, advice, and loving support as you start your dream career, consider working with me after you've finished this book.

Who This Book Is For

❋ ❋ ❋

One thing you'll learn about me if you stick around a bit is that I applaud authenticity. I want people to do work that aligns with their values. I want you to learn from the best teacher for you, find the best format for your learning style, and start your doula journey in a way that makes sense in your life.

I'll never try to convince someone that my doula trainings and coaching programs are the best for everyone. But I know for a fact they're the bomb for some folks.

For example, my birth doula training is best for people who:

- want a training that is inclusive for all people.
- believe doula work is social justice work.
- don't have the time or money to invest in an expensive doula training.
- want a low-risk way to learn a lot about the birth process and the doula role before deciding if it's the path for them.
- are curious about the spirituality, psychology, and nature of human birth.

In contrast, the doula training I took wasn't perfect for me, but it was the only one in town (and one of few in the country at that time). I started teaching for the same organization three years later and was still unsatisfied. So I created the doula training that I wished I'd had and that other doulas were asking for.

The first time I offered the doula training I created, I was brought to tears. It was authentic, so alive, so rich and full of meaning. And the response was fantastic.

I went on to study about the psychology of the pre- and perinatal period, the consciousness of babies from preconception on, attachment theory, reproductive anatomy and physiology, fetal development, reproductive endocrinology, social justice movements, anti-racism work, inclusivity, teaching methods, trauma, somatics, advocacy, and sustainability.

As I understood more and more about the human condition, I wove what I learned into my courses.

You see, your doula training is only the beginning. Once you start your new career, you too will find additional areas of interest to explore and use to specialize your work. You will inspire others to become a doula, and you can mentor them, creating a rich network of allied colleagues. You may become a trainer for a whole generation of doulas to come.

With this book, I want to create a space where people can gather and start their journey, find the path that is right for them, then dive in to learn more about what delights them along the way.

My sincere hope is that you have the magical experience I had finding myself as a doula and beyond.

Key Chapter Takeaways:

- There are many types of doulas. Aspiring doulas need help exploring the various roles, understanding the requirements for each, and discovering which one(s) are the best fit for them.

- Most doulas come to this work from a combination of personal experience, innate interest, and a desire to serve. Knowing what those are for you will help you create your path.

- Finding, and taking, a doula training is not the beginning or end of your journey. Most doulas focus in specialty areas they become interested in after they've started. You can find your niche with the services you provide, who you serve, or your unique personality or background.

A Note on Inclusive Language

I honor the gender identity of all people and don't use the pronouns she/her or he/him in this book unless I'm talking about someone who has told me their gender.

Gender identity awareness is especially important in the field of reproduction, where people who are gestating a baby may identify as a man, woman, or nonbinary—or parents may both identify as mothers, fathers, or other.

Many people in the world are gender-fluid and identify as both a man and a woman, or neither. My guideline is to not assume gender. The exceptions you will see include when I am referring to specific individuals whose pronouns I know, or when referencing someone else's words or work that used gendered language.

People have been gender-fluid, queer, transgender, gay, and lesbian as long as there have been people. This fact can be problematic for folks who were raised to think of individuals or family structures in a specific way, or whose religious upbringing has rules about what is right and wrong in gender identity and expression. You may feel yourself bristling at what you're reading; you may even want to skip this chapter or close the book and stop reading now.

If you struggle with gender diversity, I hope you will still keep reading. As a doula, you will be working with all sorts of people, and none of them will think exactly as you do. Doulas have to be open-minded to do their work well; being gender inclusive is a great place to begin.

As a doula, you must have great compassion for others, and the way to develop greater compassion is to:

- understand how individual beliefs are developed.
- identify the source of your own beliefs.
- respect that everyone has their own path to their beliefs.

Be open to understanding the complexities of gender identity and how it affects the clients you may work with in the future.

CHAPTER 3

What Is a Doula?

(If you want to skip right into the action steps to become a doula, head on over to Chapter 6. If the role of a doula is rather new to you, I invite you to take time to read this chapter and get fully oriented to doula work.)

doula noun

dou·la | \ ˈdü-lə \

plural **doulas**

: a [person] trained to provide advice, information, emotional support, and physical comfort to a [person] before, during, and just after childbirth

That's the formal definition in the Merriam-Webster online dictionary as of 12/26/2023. It's very succinct. But actually, not all doulas support birth. And there are other variations as well.

Doulas may or may not be trained. They might be certified, or not charge for their services. They may be self-employed or contract their services with an agency or organization, and serve family or friends or their entire community. Doulas may support people through reproductive events, medical events, life transitions, or the court system.

Twenty years ago, few people knew what the word *doula* meant.

Now, most people know what a doula is.

But there are so many kinds of doulas: birth, postpartum, death, full-spectrum, divorce, surgery, and more.

We need every type of doula to serve every type of family. So what is the difference between all these **types of doulas?**

And which is the one for you?

You're going to determine that in Chapters 6–9.

But for now, let's focus on the universal attributes and skills of most (if not all) doulas.

And why they are so important.

Key Principles of the Doula Role

I'd been a birth doula for ten years when I attended a death doula training. Those are two experiences at opposite ends of the spectrum, right? In the first hour, I blurted out, "That's what we do in labor!" By noon I had shared some variation of "That's just like at birth!" or "That's just like being a birth doula!" seven times. By the end of day one of a three-day training, I had repeated those phrases so many times that I knew I was annoying everyone and was going to need to shut up. But in my head for the next three days, that was my refrain: "It's just like being a birth doula!"

The core of being any kind of doula is to be of service to people in a significant—often emotionally charged and sometimes physically challenging—experience.

Think back to a challenging experience you had that didn't end up so well. A medical event, a courtroom experience, a loved one's death, a marriage. Many doulas start out wanting to help others prevent what they went through.

Imagine what that experience might have been like if you had a doula. At every turn where you felt unsure, unknowing, afraid, or pressured, someone would have been there to help you get what you needed. They couldn't have turned back the hands of time or done anything superhuman to stop the event from happening, but you would have had someone on your team. You wouldn't have been alone.

When I train doulas, I often hear new doulas say, "But isn't my job to prevent my clients from bad decisions, from making the same mistakes I made? I want to *save them* from having a bad experience or outcome."

And my response is always, "Your job is not to protect people from walking their own path. It's *their* journey. Who are you to dictate what that journey looks like? Your job is simply to offer guidance, support their decisions, and witness them along the way."

Doulas don't tell people what to do or even how to do it; they help them find their own way.

But everyone's experience is different. So how do you learn skills that can apply to everyone?

These are the **key principles of being a doula:**

- Doulas recognize that birth, postpartum, divorce, cancer, or [fill in the blank] are rites of passage that change a person emotionally, physically, and spiritually after they emerge from the experience.
- Doulas honor the inherent autonomy and respect that all people deserve when going through a challenging experience.
- Doulas acknowledge that existing systems (healthcare, legal, education, deathcare, etc.) do not serve all the emotional, physical, and spiritual needs of the people going through the experience.
- Doulas understand the intersection of racial and social oppression within these systems and how those factors impact the experiences and outcomes for marginalized people.
- Doulas believe that people are innately capable of navigating

challenging situations and know that compassion, preparation, support, and being seen make challenges more doable.

- Doulas see themselves as a bridge or stopgap measure to provide holistic support to their clients on their individual journey, while making efforts to improve the systems that are not meeting people's needs.

- Doulas understand that significant experiences are a transformative journey that can have lifelong impacts. They know how to guide a person through the transformation and the integration period afterward.

When you look at the doula role from that perspective, you may be thinking, "Wow, that's a lot. That's heavy."

Yes, it is. And that's what makes doulas so necessary in the world today.

> *"The doula role is the most profound and nuanced profession you've never heard of."*
>
> — Carrie Kenner

You'll learn more information about how to doula in your chosen field in a formal doula training, but what really makes you a doula are the key principles above.

So now we can look at the bigger picture of being a doula for any challenging experience: miscarriage, infertility, abortion, adoption, gender transition, menopause, death, marriage or wedding planning, divorce, incarceration, surgery, cancer care, psychedelic therapy—the list goes on and on.

With those key principles, a particular skill set, and specific knowledge, you can be a doula for anything!

I'm often asked if you have to be an expert in the field you practice in. No. You just need some basic knowledge for your chosen field and those magic doula skills, and you are good to go.

You don't need to know vast amounts of information—just a little bit more than your client about the systems they'll interact with, the emotional process most people experience, the physical processes they can expect, and the spiritual impact this experience may have on them. If you've already gone through the experience yourself, you probably have all the knowledge you need to begin.

Being a doula is one of the most rewarding jobs in the world, but it's more than a job—it's an identity, a calling, an act of service. It's also an entirely unique role because so few people really know **what a doula is**, much less what they do.

If you are thinking about **becoming a *birth* doula**, I have the most affordable, comprehensive, accessible **online birth doula training** around. Visit doula-training.carriekenner.com to start your birth doula today. (But I don't want you to just sign up because it's mine. Later in this book you're going to learn how to assess if being a birth doula or taking an online training is right for you.)

Primary Skills Needed to Be a Doula

Doulas uphold the key principles of being a doula using a **unique set of skills** which, when combined together, form the exquisitely nuanced role of the doula. Here they are:

- Emptying your cup of your own ideas of how the experience should go
- Developing communication skills, especially how to ask open-ended questions, listen deeply, and observe with curiosity
- Getting familiar with your client, what's important to them, and their specific desires and concerns
- Using interpersonal skills to support the relationships between your client, their chosen support people (family and/or friends), the professional staff, the system(s) they're operating within, and you
- Translating your client's seemingly unrelated past experiences into

what could be helpful for the new journey ahead (for example, applying what they learned from being in grad school to how to prepare for birth)

- Being emotionally and physically open and present for your clients
- Accessing intuitive skills, specifically how to "read" a room, notice shifting energy, and watch what is unfolding around you
- Identifying the physical, emotional, mental, spiritual, and social terrain of the life situation you are working in
- Understanding the systems you'll be working in (for example, healthcare, adoption, legal, financial, deathcare)
- Being familiar with the facilities you'll be working in (for example, hospitals, courts, prisons)
- Knowing comfort measures and strategies for coping with physical pain, if appropriate
- Recognizing the physical and medical conditions that arise in your field, and options for addressing them
- Appreciating the mental health impacts of your chosen field
- Considering holistic care for your clients and yourself
- Keeping your personal stories and opinions to yourself
- Sharing allegorical stories as a means to educate and offer options
- Advocating for people in a way that doesn't take away their power
- Asking for consent before offering ideas or an intervention
- Networking and accessing resources for information, family support, and community services
- Operating from a trauma-informed perspective
- Being diplomatic while changing the world

As you can see, the above list doesn't include much about how to do a double-hip squeeze in labor, how to file for divorce, or how to dress a body for a funeral. All that stuff is the technical support you provide on top of the key competencies above.

I am one hundred percent certain that whatever field you are interested in, you're already learning about it. You're probably watching people in your field on YouTube or have a library of podcasts or have checked out a dozen websites on the topic.

Way to prepare!

CHAPTER 4

The History and Breadth of the Doula Movement

The word *doula* is a Greek word that means "female servant," and was adopted by anthropologist Dana Raphael in the 1970s in her book *The Tender Gift: Breastfeeding*. The doula role was defined as a woman serving women, replacing the historical family and community support people would have received in traditional communities before, during, and after birth.

The modern doula movement originated around the event of childbirth but has now grown to encompass all aspects of reproduction, other significant life transitions, and medical care.

The doula movement that focused on the birth and postpartum period was started primarily by white, middle class, middle-aged women who viewed their doula work more as a hobby than a career. They understood the significance of pregnant and birthing people being separated from their familiar support networks during birth and postpartum, but they didn't understand the additional impact this separation had on oppressed and marginalized people.

This is important to understand because the founders of that doula movement defined how the doula role was designed to function, based on their vantage point. It was passive, woman-centered, attainable only to those with privilege, and not considered a profession.

It wasn't until the 2000s that white doula organizations began to listen to their marginalized colleagues and acknowledge disparities in birth outcomes for people of color and the impacts of systemic racism and trauma on oppressed and marginalized people.

Many changes have occurred in the doula movement to make it more accessible, impactful, relevant, and oriented to systemic change, but its origins continue to plague the doula role with outdated and limited visions of how to provide support and empowerment.

When I became a doula, I saw the doula movement as an opportunity to support people who were often disrespected and marginalized in birth, and as a way for entrepreneurial-minded people to find work they loved that could provide them with financial freedom.

One of the key factors for success as a doula is *authenticity*. This is one field where you get rewarded for being yourself.

We have a motto in the birth world, but it applies to all fields: *A doula for every person who wants one.* We make it really clear that no one doula is the right doula for every person who wants one. Besides being physically impossible, it's not respectful either.

A client might want a doula who is like them—of the same age, culture, religion, and ethnicity. At first, there were very few doulas from marginalized communities. That is finally changing. As a white doula, I make sure doulas who come from privileged backgrounds learn what life is like for oppressed people and help them find resources so that anyone in their community can find a doula they resonate with.

But I also never make assumptions about who a person might want as their doula. A client might want someone older or younger, energetic or calming, take-charge or more of a witness. When I was younger, I was more like a peer to my clients. As I got older, I was more like a mother. I attracted different clients over time, and how I liked to work as a doula changed too.

I'll not only help you figure out what kind of doula role is best for you and where to get trained, I'll help you determine who you are and how you want to be as a doula—and who you'd like to work with the most to find your sweet spot.

Know thyself, be yourself.

Over the years, my greatest delight has come from answering questions of aspiring doulas, plugging in to their excitement and dreams, and coaching them to step on the path and go for it. What they have asked for and needed has inspired the next course or program I created.

Everything that I've developed has come from a place of listening to what doulas said they wanted. A doula training that addressed racial and social justice? Check. A retreat to fill your soul so you could return to your family and clients re-energized? Check. A doula training that is all online? Check.

My own struggles to start and grow a business when no one else was doing it drove me to create business courses and, ultimately, my business coaching program.

I fulfilled my dream to own my own business, to work with families at birth, to make my living doing something I love, and to make the world a better place, one birth, one family, one doula at a time.

I'm not the only one who's achieved these results. Here are some examples from the people I've worked with.

Doula Story #1: Breaking the Glass Ceiling

Alice and I met right after our birth doula training. Alice was a single mom who intended to make her living as a doula; I was trying to replace my corporate income. The most experienced and well-known birth doula in town didn't need to make a living at her work; her husband was a doctor. Her doula fee did not create a liveable wage. And many of the doulas in the area considered doula work a hobby and didn't want or need to get paid for it. That was fine for them, but what about people like Alice and me who wanted this important work to be their livelihood?

Alice and I approached the queen bee doula and explained that the doula role was no longer a hobby. We talked about how work that was primarily *for* women, done primarily *by* women, was often undervalued, and asked her to please raise her rates to send a message that this work was important and valuable. Otherwise, our rates were going to surpass hers, which felt presumptuous and disrespectful.

She gave us her blessing to raise our rates, and in the next four years, the going rate for birth doulas in our area doubled and career doulas flourished.

❋ ❋ ❋

Doula Story #2: Making the Leap

Carol joined my doula business coaching program. She was a full-time nanny but wanted to make the leap to full-time birth doula work. She developed strategies to market for more clients and created a plan for when she could make the switch.

Her goal: Quit her nanny job.

To do this, Carol made a plan. She would have one month of income saved up + have two clients booked for the next three months + get on two providers' referral lists. Then, she could quit.

She would try to fill another one to two clients in the next three months, but she had that financial cushion if she didn't.

By the end of the program, Carol had quit her nanny job and was a full-time doula.

She has since attended 550 births and recently received an award for being of service to the most families in a community-based doula program.

Doula Story #3: Changing the Face of Doula Business

Rachel and Vivian were two up-and-coming birth and postpartum doulas in my doula training. They had a great sense for business and had a business plan before they even stepped into the classroom. After they completed the training, they formed a partnership, started charging the top rate for doulas immediately (which was not common practice), and within the year had a thriving practice that supported *both* of them financially.

They consulted with other doulas interested in forming a partnership and promoted a model of sustainability that was unusual in the doula community at that time.

Eight years later, they both decided to move on to other professions. When most doulas leave the field, they just stop doing the work and close their business. Rachel and Vivian *sold* their business for a profit to two doulas just starting out, gave them the jumpstart they needed, and left a legacy for alternative ways doulas could structure their business.

Doula Story #4: An Agency to Weather a Cancer Diagnosis

Janice trained with me as a birth doula. She was a single mom to a young son and was so inspired by the doula care she had received at her birth that she wanted to become that kind of support for others. It was hard to be on call for births with a young child, so she also trained as a postpartum doula and was able to schedule childcare more readily for that work. Janice ran a successful birth and postpartum doula business through the pregnancy and birth of her second son, and through the pregnancy of her third.

Then, the unexpected happened. Janice's third son was diagnosed with cancer at the age of two. The treatment would be long and taxing on the whole family. There was no way Janice could tend to families full-time when she had so much to do to care for her own.

Janice didn't want all of her doula skills to go to waste, and in between her son's treatment cycles, she was able to work as a doula. So she started a postpartum doula agency that would continue to attract new clients and where she could send doulas out in her stead. She used her knowledge of marketing, client management, and business savvy (which she learned in my business coaching program) to brand a new business, with the focus of creating a village of parents and support. She contracted with a team of doulas who enjoyed more flexibility with night or day shifts and built-in backup than they could create on their own. And when she was at the hospital with her son for weeks on end, she could still generate an income from her agency.

Doula Story #5: From Birth to Death Doula to Postpartum Doula

Sarah was a successful birth doula for decades, but as she entered her 50s, the on-call lifestyle caught up with her. She went back to school to get a master's degree in public health and worked in healthcare administration for the next decade, but the call to be with families at the end of life tugged her back to one-on-one care.

Sarah got a job in hospice that was shift-based and reliable, but it didn't allow her the personal relationship-building she thrived on as a doula. She loved working with families and individuals at the end of life, but the on-call nature of being a death doula was daunting because she was now moving well into her sixties.

By this point in her life, Sarah had two adult children who lived nearby and was grandmother to five. She had been able to provide live-in support to her kids when they had a new baby. She recognized the similarity in family dynamics and shifting identities that occurred at the end of life and postpartum. So Sarah combined her skills as a doula and her knowledge of babies, families, and postpartum to become a postpartum doula.

Sarah took advantage of the fact that many new parents live far from their parents. Some people really want a "grandma" nearby, and as an experienced real-life Grammie, Sarah was a great fit. Now, she could schedule clients during the day, be with her family in the evenings, and offer night time shifts if she wanted to. She gained control over her lifestyle, sleep, and health.

CHAPTER 5

What's Stopping You?

Like I said, in 2001, if you wanted to become a doula, you had to carve out two to four full days to attend an in-person training. If you had a job, you had to get (unpaid) time off. If you had kids, you needed childcare. If it wasn't in your hometown, add on the cost for travel and accommodations.

Trainings back then were pretty basic and didn't include how to start a business at all.

Lucky for you, all that has changed.

Now, though, you have an entirely different set of problems: too many options. Online or in-person, two days or nine months, with a group or work at your own pace... With so many variations, it can be hard to know where to start.

After twenty years of working as a doula and training doulas, I've learned a few things. Things you can only learn by doing, observing, and coaching.

I want to share with you what I've seen in my twenty-year career for two reasons:

1. So that you can learn from others' concerns and avoid making mistakes yourself

2. To show you exactly why I think my process is so badass

I think you'll find a tremendous amount of value in seeing things through the eyes of an experienced doula. Here's my summary of the obstacles most doulas face when starting out:

Issue #1: There are so many doula roles. My framework helps you figure out if being a doula—and what kind of doula—is right for you.

Just because you love pregnant people or babies doesn't mean you can be a birth doula. Being a birth doula requires being on-call, being able to drop whatever you're doing at a moment's notice, and being okay with blood and poop. Not you? But still love babies and pregnancy? Become an antenatal, abortion, adoption, or postpartum doula.

In Chapter 6, I'm going to outline all the doula roles, what they do, where and when they do it, who they primarily work with, and so much more, so you know all your options.

Issue #2: There are so many training choices. My framework helps you assess doula trainings to find the best one for you.

Not all doula trainings are created equal. They may not be as comprehensive as you expect, or cover both doula skills and business skills, or provide material in the way you learn best.

You may have to choose between how the training is delivered, the charisma of the trainer, the focus of the content, and the cost. Don't worry. They don't all have to line up perfectly. You can take a low-cost training that includes the information you want but isn't with your ideal trainer. Later, you can take trainings from your dream trainer and soak up their knowledge.

In Chapters 11–14, I'm going to help you determine the best kind of training for *you* and how to assess trainings for their features, such as method of delivery, time requirements, length, support, cost, and more. Then, I'll help you prioritize what's most important for you in your training, so you have realistic expectations of what your training can provide and common pitfalls to watch out for—like what the hidden messages are in how a doula training markets itself, or the key phrases that tell you a training is not comprehensive.

Issue #3: You don't have a lot of money or time to invest in training. My framework shows you how to determine the real cost of a doula training and inquire about payment options.

There's the cost of the training and the cost of *attending* the training. If you have to travel, miss time from work, buy extra books or supplies, or take many months to complete it, your training may not be the bonanza you expected. Remember, your doula training is not the end-all be-all of your education. Find one that meets your basic needs and know you'll learn more after that.

In Chapter 15, I'll also show you how to budget the time and money for your training to fit where you are at in life now.

Issue #4: You worry you'll take a training and find out it's not the right role for you. My framework will help you become confident in your choices.

Unfortunately, doula training organizations are like lots of other businesses—they want you as a client even if they're not the best fit for you. Their sales page may be beautiful and their course content may check all the boxes, but how do you know what you need if you're not a doula yet?

It's like you need a doula to help you become a doula—that's me!

If you complete all the assessments in this book, you'll have a crystal clear idea of which doula role is a good fit for where you are now, as well as other doula roles you might want to pursue in the future, when your life circumstances may be different. You'll have looked at a few possible training options and know how to select one that meets the majority of your requirements. You'll feel confident that you are making the best choice for you in this moment.

Issue #5: How will you find clients? What's the job market like? My framework tells you how to assess your local market, the going rate, and research opportunities to start your business.

You may have heard many stories of people getting trained to be a doula and then never actually doula-ing. This is all too common and doesn't need to be so!

I'm going to show you what to research *before* you invest in your training. Is there a demand in your area? What's the going rate for your type of doula? And how do you attract clients and get them to hire you?

Chapter 17 was built with this in mind. Knowing this process will give you the confidence, inspiration, and motivation to pursue your doula career.

Issue #6: You worry about licensing, certification, and insurance. My framework helps you find out what you need to know about your doula field, current trends, and future possibilities.

Starting a new career can be so confusing. And this is one area your doula training may not solve for you. Because regulations and laws vary in different jurisdictions (city, county, state, province, country, etc.) and because they *change*, you cannot rely on someone else to feed you this information.

I'm going to show you how to do your own research on business structures, professional requirements, liabilities, where to look to get answers, and the difference between standards, protocols, certifications, regulations, laws, and more.

Knowing all this information now—before you train to become a doula—is going to make all the difference in your doula career. You're going to know from the beginning that:

- you are on the right path.
- you are properly prepared.
- you know what to expect ahead.

Sounds like a perfect journey! Ready to get started? The next sections of this book will walk you through the Become a Doula framework step-by-step.

Part 2: The *Become a Doula Framework* covers these three points:

Point #1: Too many times, people want to be a doula without knowing what it entails. This book will give you a realistic understanding of multiple doula roles to find the one you can succeed in.

Point #2: People spend thousands of dollars on doula trainings that don't provide what they need in a format they can digest. I'll show you how to assess and choose a training that you'll actually learn from and complete.

Point #3: For decades, doulas have struggled to create a successful career because they didn't know they'd have to start a business or they didn't know how to. I wrote Part 4: Preparing for a Doula Career in this book to change all that.

Part 2

The Become a Doula Framework

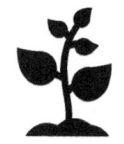

CHAPTER 6

Step 1: What Kind of Doula Role Are You Interested In?

This section is all about matching *you* with your perfect doula role. We're going to look at your specific areas of interest, learn about twenty-six different doula roles, and see which ones will best fit with your lifestyle. But before we dive into all of that, let's see how ready you are for your new career as a doula.

Starting a new career, or shifting from one to another, will vary in difficulty based on your financial situation, your lifestyle flexibility, and your capacity to learn new things at this stage in your life. None of the assessments in this book will tell you you can or can't do anything. They're all designed to get you thinking about certain things, reflect for yourself on what they mean, and offer solutions for moving forward.

So, let's start with the Career Readiness Assessment. This is a high-level look at where you are in life right now, so you can realistically prepare for becoming a doula. Even if you don't have a "career" per se, it will help you determine what might help you get ready to learn the skills you need as a doula.

CAREER READINESS ASSESSMENT

The following questions are designed to get you thinking about what you might need to have in place before you transition to a new career as a doula. They look at your overall financial picture, your preference for starting out in a new field, and your capacity (time and energy) to learn new subject matter.

This questionnaire does not intend to cause self-judgment or raise concerns yet often when people complete it, they start conjuring up scenarios in their minds of what their answers predict for their future. Don't worry about coming up with solutions to any complications you are imagining. Just be aware of your needs for now.

Financial Flexibility

*Choose the **one** statement that most closely fits your current situation:*

☐	I do not have to support myself financially, OR I provide my sole support or contribute to my family's financial well-being and I have 3+ months of savings I can live off.	Score 5
☐	I am willing and able to reduce my income if necessary as I start out in a new career.	Score 3
☐	I provide the sole financial support for myself and have no savings	Score 1
☐	I am able to earn money at my current job AND take on new work as a doula while I make the transition from one job to another.	Score 4
☐	I contribute to the financial well-being of my household and have no savings	Score 2

Your financial flexibility score: _____

What your score means:
1 = You can start training for your doula role now but will need savings or a plan in place for someone else to support you as you transition to doula work.
2 = Decide if your family can survive without your current income when you transition to doula work; if not, reduce your expenses and/or save a few months of income for making the change
3-4 = Make a financial transition plan, with goals and milestones, to track your doula business growth. Have a backup plan for additional income if you don't hit your targets in the first 2 months.
5 = Dive in!

Step 1: What Kind of Doula Role Are You Interested In?

Career Flexibility	
*Choose the **one** statement that most closely fits your current situation:*	
☐ I am willing to sacrifice my sense of competence and identity from my current career	Score 5
☐ Even though I love my existing life, I am willing to change and adjust it to accommodate my future doula career.	Score 5
☐ I am able to start AND finish new things easily	Score 4
☐ I am able to work independently	Score 3
☐ I am able to be self-motivated	Score 3
Your career flexibility score:	_____

What your score means:
0-6 - Choose a doula role that is closely related to your current work and plan to work for a doula agency if one exists in your area.
7-14 You have many of the characteristics of someone who can start a new career and be motivated to run their own business. For areas that you did not score in, consider finding a mentor or business coach to help you gain skills and confidence.
15-22 You are well poised to start a new business and career.

Adjustment Flexibility	
*Choose the **one** statement that most closely fits your current situation:*	
☐ I love my existing life and don't want to change it; I want a doula career that fits in it easily	Score 1
☐ I love my existing life but am willing to modify it; I want a doula career that won't require a total adjustment	Score 2
☐ I love my existing life but am willing to change it; I am willing to adjust a lot to accommodate my future doula career	Score 3
Your adjustment flexibility score:	_____

What your score means:
1 = Choose a doula role that is schedule-based and where the typical activities can fit around your existing lifestyle.
2 = Choose a doula role that is schedule-based.
3 = Sounds like you can pursue any doula role you are interested in.

Learning Flexibility	
*Choose the **one** statement that most closely fits your current situation:*	
☐ I'm new to this field but I am willing to learn new information and skills to become a doula, AND I have the time to do so.	Score 5
☐ I love learning new things but am limited on how much time/energy I have to learn new things to become a doula	Score 2
☐ I have some knowledge already in the field I'd like to become a doula but limited time to learn more	Score 3
☐ I have a lot of knowledge already in the field I'd like to become a doula	Score 4
Your learning flexibility score:	_____
What your score means: 1-2 = Allow yourself extra time to train as a doula, and be sure to "budget" your training time into your calendar. 3-4 = Find the doula training you need and get started!	

Access this and all other forms online at https://doula-training.carriekenner.com/doula-assessment-forms-book

I hope the assessment was helpful for looking a bit into your future. Now, let's talk about what that future might look like in your role as a doula.

A doula typically works with people preparing for a significant life experience. Usually, the event they are planning for has a physical or emotional component to it; often both.

A doula:

- helps their client explore and clarify their beliefs and values about the event they are facing.
- provides them with information about what to expect and skills to help them navigate the situation.
- accompanies them during the event to provide emotional and/or physical support, advocacy, and witness, if appropriate.
- helps them process and integrate their experience afterward.

Here's a list of things the modern doula does and doesn't do:

Step 1: What Kind of Doula Role Are You Interested In?

THINGS DOULAS DO	THINGS DOULAS DON'T DO
Provide non-judgmental support and leave decisions to their client.	Tell clients what they should do, or make decisions for them.
Provide information about the event they are facing, typical practices, and what to expect.	Provide medical or clinical care or legal advice, make diagnoses, prescribe treatment, or make specific recommendations, unless the doula is trained and legally able to do so.
Advocate for the client's wishes based on prior conversations, requests, and/or in discussions during the event.	Speak for their client without the client's permission or request.
Encourage and facilitate conversations between the client and their care providers or other professionals.	Tell clinical staff what their client wants, unless the client has asked the doula to help with communication or the client is not being listened to.
Support clients with decision-making.	Make decisions for their client.
Amplify their client's voice if they are not being listened to.	Allow their client to be coerced or violated without intervening.
Provide referrals to other care providers.	Do things outside their scope of practice or skill set and knowledge base.
Be on call for events that can't be scheduled (such as birth or death).	Make themselves unavailable during their on-call time.
Provide continuous care (more on this later).	Leave clients without support during their experience, limit their client's access without advance notice, or refuse to provide backup care.
Hold their clients as their primary responsibility, and hold their client's information in strict confidence.	Share information about their clients.

THINGS DOULAS DO	THINGS DOULAS DON'T DO
Stay up-to-date about specific practices, policies, or regulations in their community, recent research, and network in their community.	Work in isolation.
Become an ambassador for doula care in their larger community.	

Now, let's look at twenty-six specific doula roles that you can explore.

I'm going to organize the various doula roles into three major categories:

1. Reproduction
2. Life Transitions
3. Medical

Even though they are categorized like this, there is also some overlap. For example, a gender-transition doula is supporting someone through a life transition that may also include medical care. Or an infertility doula may have been supporting someone through assisted reproductive technology—a medical process—and is now helping them navigate adoption, a life transition.

It doesn't matter how I've categorized them—the most important thing is for you to think about what areas interest you. Complete the Interest Assessment to see what you find out about yourself, and then use those findings with the Doula-bility Calculator in Chapter 9.

Step 1: What Kind of Doula Role Are You Interested In?

INTEREST ASSESSMENT

This assessment is designed to raise your awareness of topics or interests you naturally gravitate toward. You do not need to have experience, education, or training in any of these things to be interested in them. I just want you to see for yourself where you might be an eager doula.

On a scale of 0 - 10 (0 = no interest, 10 = most interest), enter your interest number for each item.

INTEREST SCORE	AREA OF INTEREST	CODE
	GENDER	**CODE**
	Women's issues	W
	Men's issues	M
	Gender/transgender issues	G
	MEDICAL	**CODE**
	Women's health	W
	Men's health	M
	Transgender health	G
	Sexual health	X
	Holistic/alternative health	H
	Nutrition/diet	N
	Chronic illness	IL
	Cancer	CA
	Surgery	S
	Psychedelic therapy	PS
	AGE	**CODE**
	Babies and infants	B
	Teens	T
	Adults	L
	Menopause	MP
	Elders	E

	REPRODUCTION	CODE
	Menstruation	R
	Birth control	BC
	Fertility and preconception	F
	Abortion	A
	Miscarriage	MC
	Surrogacy	SR
	Pregnancy and birth	PB
	Postpartum	PP
	LIFE TRANSITIONS	**CODE**
	Puberty/coming of age	T
	Gender transition	G
	Parenthood	PA
	Menopause	MP
	Marriage/wedding	MR
	Adoption	O
	Pets (adoption, training, or loss)	P
	Divorce	DV
	Court/legal cases	C
	Incarceration	I
	Grief and Loss	GR
	Dementia	E
	Death/End of life/Hospice	D

⬇
For any scores higher than a 5, transfer the CODE to the Doula-bility Calculator in Chapter 9

Access this and all other forms online at https://doula-training.carriekenner.com/doula-assessment-forms-book

Step 1: What Kind of Doula Role Are You Interested In?

Twenty-Six Different Types of Doulas (and Counting)

Remember, all doulas are professional companions who provide advocacy, knowledge, and support. Unless otherwise noted, they do not provide technical (i.e. clinical or legal) services or advice.

Reproduction Doulas

Menstruation

Menstruation or Menarche (onset of menstruation) doulas support menstruating people with their menstrual cycles. They may provide information, physical aids, and emotional or energetic support to help people have empowering and comfortable experiences with their cycles. They can create rituals for those just starting to menstruate, for each cycle, or for the cessation of menstruation (see menopause doulas below).

This work is recommended and helpful for people who are just beginning to menstruate, have difficult menstrual cycles, or who have PMS, endometriosis, or other medical conditions.

Birth Control

Birth control doulas help people navigate the myriad choices for preventing pregnancy. They offer information on birth control options (barrier, hormonal, pharmaceutical, herbal, and others), provide emotional and educational support for people as they choose or transition between birth control options, help clients chart their menstrual cycles, and facilitate access to contraception services and care. A birth control doula may help clients discuss their concerns and priorities, accompany people to healthcare appointments, provide fertility awareness lessons, and interpret their menstrual charts.

Preconception

Preconception doulas support people who are planning a pregnancy. Preconception support can include emotional, physical, nutritional, lifestyle, and spiritual preparation for pregnancy and welcoming a child into their life. It may also include fertility/infertility support (see fertility/infertility doulas below). Fertility awareness, evidence-based information, menstrual-cycle tracking, lifestyle assessments, and relationship-coaching may also be a part of the preconception doula's role.

Fertility/Infertility

A fertility doula accompanies people through their fertility journey and provides educational and emotional support during the preconception-to-conception stage. Fertility doulas help their clients navigate the medical maze of fertility treatments and reproductive technology by providing information on options, non-judgemental support, and holistic approaches to support fertility treatments. They can make lifestyle suggestions, provide evidence-based information, and teach mindfulness and relaxation techniques to assist the process. Fertility doulas may accompany clients to medical appointments or be on hand to process experiences afterward.

Abortion

An abortion doula provides physical and emotional support to a patient before, during, and after the abortion process. Their goal is to complement the medical care, tune in to whatever the patients' needs are, support their emotional and psychological needs, and help them be as comfortable as possible during the process. Abortion doulas make sure a client knows their options, gets the information they need to make decisions, advocates for them, and provides coping support during the procedure. These doulas are also trained in trauma-informed care and reproductive rights as part of their role.

Miscarriage

A miscarriage doula is someone who provides information and support to people who experience pregnancy loss (typically at any gestation in pregnancy). Their support may include listening to clients' experiences, providing information on options, advocating for their client's preferences, and providing in-person support during the process. They may take pictures, coordinate support with friends and family, lead letting-go rituals, and attend followup medical visits. They provide emotional and mental support through grief coaching and are trauma-informed.

Surrogacy

Surrogacy doulas can provide support to either/both surrogates and intended parents during meetings, and make sure participants know their options for pregnancy, birth, and postpartum. They can help with birth planning, provide labor support, and help with transitioning the baby. After birth, surrogacy doulas can provide postpartum support to intended parents or surrogates to ensure their medical and emotional needs are being met, and help process the experience. Surrogacy doulas may be hired to support just the surrogate, the intended parents, or both.

Antepartum/Antenatal (aka Bed Rest)

Antepartum doulas offer support to families that are experiencing a difficult pregnancy, physical restrictions, or other challenging conditions. These doulas provide companionship, information, options, coping strategies, household support, care coordination, and birth preparation. Emotional support is also key, as clients may need to process fears, frustration, and physical discomfort. Antenatal doulas often support high-risk pregnancies, teen parents, medical complications, morning sickness, or others who need extra support during pregnancy.

Birth

Birth doulas support people during pregnancy, the birth process, and early postpartum. They meet with their clients during their pregnancy to learn about their wishes and preferences, teach them about the birth process and what to expect, join them in labor to provide emotional and physical support, help them make decisions during labor, stay with them as long as it takes for their baby to be born, support them in the first few hours after birth, and check in on the family in the few weeks after birth. In general, birth doulas need to be on call from the time their clients are 36 to 42 weeks pregnant, be able to join them within an hour of being called, and be prepared to stay for up to forty-eight hours.

Contrary to popular myth, birth doulas support any kind of birth (natural, medicated, or cesarean), in all places (home, birth center, and hospital), with any care provider (midwives and doctors). They don't have to have given birth themselves, and they range in age from teens to people in their seventies.

Postpartum

Postpartum doulas support new families in the first weeks or months after having a baby. The postpartum support most new parents experience is the one to two days they spend in the hospital after giving birth, and then they are sent home utterly alone. Family and friends might be waiting to support them at home, but these helpers are often filled with opinions, judgment, potentially outdated information, and visions of holding the baby while the new parents take care of their household. What new parents really need is household support, meals, evidence-based information, kind, listening ears, lots of space to learn as they go, and someone who wants to honor their wishes

Postpartum doulas come to the family's home a few times a week after the baby is born, and typically spend about four hours helping with laundry; food preparation; organizing; infant feeding; infant care (such as bathing, soothing, or babywearing); listening; facilitating conversations between the parents and other support people; providing tips for comfort; holding the baby so parents can nap, shower, or have a bit of time alone; and light housekeeping such as watering plants, vacuuming, and washing dishes.

Postpartum doulas also provide overnight care to help parents get optimal sleep. The doula will stay with the baby while it sleeps and bring the baby to the parents for feeding during the night, or handle feeding duties if the parents do not want to be disturbed. They may also provide minimal household support while the baby sleeps.

Life Transition Doulas

Menarche

A menarche (onset of menstruation) doula supports a person as they approach the beginning of their menstruating years. They may help a person prepare emotionally and physically for the beginning of menstruation, provide information, offer spiritual and emotional support, and suggest practices to support this time of life and their future cycles. They may also create individual or community rituals to celebrate the coming of menstruation as a rite of passage.

Gender and/or Gender Transition

A gender doula supports an individual—and their family and friends, if desired—as they explore their gender identity; establish their gender identity in all aspects of life; and help them navigate legal, educational, or medical systems. They may help facilitate conversations with family members; act as an advocate in many situations; walk them through the process of changing their name, for example; and support them emotionally and spiritually through any challenges they are facing. Gender doulas support people wherever they are in their gender identity journey.

A gender transition doula supports people before, during, and after the process of physical or medical transitions. They may help them access medical care, attend medical visits, understand medication options and side effects, serve as an advocate within the healthcare system, attend medical visits, help with decision-making, and recommend resources.

Marriage and/or Wedding

A marriage doula provides emotional, spiritual, and practical support to a couple as they prepare for a life of marriage. They may provide premarital counseling, planning, and information sessions that help them clarify their intentions and build trust and resilience in their relationship. They facilitate conversations and expectations with family and friends as they approach their wedding, and help blended families communicate and unite.

Wedding doulas help clients navigate the wedding-planning industry. They help them know their options, articulate their dreams and desires, prepare and guide them through the challenges and frustrations of the planning process, and support them in making mindful decisions. Along the way, they provide stress-relieving tools.

Wedding doulas may help with logistics and communication leading up to the wedding, and may attend the wedding to provide emotional and spiritual support to keep them focused on enjoying the day. A wedding doula will help manage logistical details and help the day go smoothly. Some marriage doulas may also work as wedding doulas and wedding officiants.

Adoption

Adoption doulas specialize in adoptions. For newborn adoptions, they provide information, education, guidance, support, and resources during the pregnancy, through the birth, and early postpartum. Their goal is to ensure a smooth transition for the birthing person, the baby, and the adopting family.

An adoption doula may provide typical birth doula support to the birthing person, immediate postpartum coordination for all parties, postpartum support for the adopting family, and education, emotional support, logistical support, and resources to all involved. They may work with both parties or just one.

They may also provide support to families for older-child adoptions by helping them navigate the legal process, prepare their household, access resources, and support relationships and family integration.

Pet Adoption or Loss

Pet doulas support people with pets in many ways. While most pet doulas work with families whose pets are nearing end-of-life, they can also help any family with pet-related transitions. As with any doula, they provide information, options, support, and presence. For end-of-life situations, they may assist with veterinary care, ceremonies, burial, and processing grief. For new pets, pet doulas come into the home to help families prepare for bringing a new pet into the family, or bringing a new baby into a family with pets. They may teach skills, translate pet behaviors, provide resources, and develop strategies for a smooth transition.

Menopause

Menopause doulas help clients going through the very individual experience of perimenopause or menopause transition. They provide information on the biology, hormonal changes, and physical and nutritional changes of menopause; guidance, tips, and resources; and emotional support, comfort strategies, and options to discuss with their care provider.

Menopause doulas serve as an adjunct to their client's health care team, such as physicians, nutritionists, and health coaches. They often refer clients to these service providers and help them navigate medical care that is appropriate and tailored for people during menopause.

Because menopause can last many years, regular check-ins to assess the client's well-being and providing resources are key doula responsibilities.

They may facilitate conversations and awareness, put an end to many myths about menopause, and empower clients with a customized transition strategy.

Divorce

Divorce is one of the most stressful experiences of life. Divorce doulas help clients navigate this complex emotional, legal, and financial journey. They educate clients about the various types of divorce, and develop a plan to minimize the emotional distress and financial upheaval that divorce can cause.

During divorce, people are typically in high-stress mode. Divorce doulas help reduce stress to protect their client's nervous system and prevent their judgment from being clouded, so clients can make clear decisions. They also help clients know what to expect in the divorce process, and help them prioritize, organize, and prepare for deadlines and meetings. They may attend meetings with their clients to offer emotional support and advocacy.

A divorce doula helps clients identify what they want their post-divorce life to look like and how to get there, from where they'll live, to jobs and finances, to co-parenting. Divorce doulas help empower clients as they find their way to a new future.

Court or Judicial System

Similar to a divorce doula, a court doula supports people through the daunting task of entering the courts or judicial system. Court doulas meet with clients and/or their families to educate them on the legal process they are entering, how it works, and what to expect. They provide information and resources to make decisions, and provide emotional support as they navigate through their trial. There is currently no training for this doula role. Most people working in this role have a background in the judicial system and want to help mitigate the stress and confusion many people experience when entering the legal system.

Incarceration

An incarceration doula helps families with a loved one in jail or prison navigate the prison system. They provide logistical information on prison life, visitation, how to stay in contact with someone who is incarcerated, and more. They provide emotional support and resources to help families access financial support, legal needs, and mental health. They help families prepare for release and provide suggestions for welcome-home rituals, emotional processing, integration, and support to avoid post-incarceration syndrome. There is currently no training for this doula role. Most people working in this capacity have experienced loved ones in prison or incarceration and want to help ease the journey for others.

Grief

A grief doula supports people through the process of grief following a loss or major life change. Grief may be the result of death, miscarriage, divorce, a medical condition, the end of a friendship or significant relationship, loss of a career, family estrangement, and other important transitions. They provide emotional support, explain what to expect in the grief process, offer tools for coping and processing, and provide resources. Grief doulas may also help design rituals, coordinate logistical support, provide spiritual guidance, and offer body-based support such as energy work, movement, and massage.

Many grief doulas are also end-of-life or death doulas, but the grief role focuses specifically on the emotional aftermath of a loss.

Dementia

Dementia doulas help people and their families navigate living with dementia. They provide nonclinical logistical support, such as coordinating medical care, meal services, occupational therapy, and medication management. They offer emotional support and respite resources for families as needs change.

They can also assist in finding home- and community-support services, offer information on options, attend meetings as a support person, and serve as an on-call point person.

End of Life

An end-of-life doula helps individuals and families prepare for death. Their work can start as soon as someone receives a prognosis of death, a few weeks or months before someone dies, and proactively for those who want to prepare for the inevitable.

End-of-life doulas provide emotional, informational, practical, and spiritual support to their clients. They can help with wills, estates, or legacy planning, and can enhance traditional medical care by offering an additional layer of support. They meet with clients regularly to provide information and options, answer questions, listen, facilitate conversations, and support decision-making. They may be at the bedside during the dying process, and may be involved in preparing a body for final disposition.

Many end-of-life doulas are also death or grief doulas, but this role specifically focuses on supporting individuals and families as they approach death.

Death

Death doulas help individuals and families prepare for the dying process. They provide information, options, emotional and spiritual support, facilitate conversations, and support decision-making. A death doula helps a dying person and their family members speak openly and honestly about dying by having conversations that many people find uncomfortable.

Death doulas accompany their clients through the dying process. They are at the bedside providing emotional and logistical support, and often assist family members with preparing the body for final disposition, designing or leading rituals, and helping to plan memorial or funeral services.

Many death doulas are also end-of-life doulas or grief doulas, but this role specifically focuses on supporting individuals and families through the active process of death and the immediate aftermath of preparing the body for final disposition and memorial or funeral services.

Medical Doulas

Cancer

Cancer doulas bridge the gap between the medical and emotional aspects of a cancer diagnosis and treatment. They help individuals and families navigate the healthcare system, understand treatment options, coordinate medical care, and manage home, work, and finances. Their focus is on physical, emotional, mental, and spiritual health during their cancer journey.

Cancer doulas are a combination of personal guide and patient advocate. They typically meet with clients in their home, coordinate communication with their healthcare team, and may attend medical visits with them as well. They make sure clients are informed and educated, are listened to and their choices are respected, and are connected with available resources.

Cancer doulas typically have a background in healthcare, a personal experience with cancer, or are involved with cancer support organizations.

Illness

Illness doulas guide clients through diagnosis, treatment options, medical care, and lifestyle changes after a chronic illness is diagnosed. They provide emotional, informational, and logistical support, often by attending medical visits; surgery prep; and follow-up care. Illness doulas ensure that clients are informed of all treatment options, assist them with decision-making, help them have medical directives in place, and make sure their wishes are followed. They may coordinate insurance and billing issues, communication among the healthcare team and family members, and assist with accommodations their client may need.

Illness doulas often have a background in healthcare or a personal experience of chronic illness. Their goal is to reduce feelings of shame, grief, loneliness, and overwhelm of newly diagnosed illnesses.

Psychedelic Therapy

A psychedelic therapy doula assists clients with the preparation and integration of a psychedelic medicine journey. They provide information on what to expect, elicit their client's desires and goals for their experience, and guide them with emotional and spiritual preparation for an altered state of consciousness. Psychedelic therapy doulas typically attend the journey, helping with physical needs, providing a grounding presence, and coordinating with the professional guide. After the journey, they help their client integrate their experience.

CHAPTER 7

Step 2: Your Lifestyle Assessment

To be successful at any job, you need these three things:

1. An interest or passion in the job
2. A job that's a good fit for your personality and lifestyle
3. The skills to do the job well

You just learned about your **interests** in the last chapter.

This chapter will help you understand your **current lifestyle and preferences** to identify the doula role that will be the best fit for you (or help you make adjustments in your life for other doula roles).

(You'll learn about the **skills** you'll need as a doula in Chapter 10.)

Are you able to be on call for birth or death? Are you comfortable interacting with big systems like healthcare or judicial courts? Do you like working with families or individuals?

This is just a sampling of the questions you're going to ask yourself in this chapter.

So let's dive in and take a look at your current lifestyle and preferences.

LIFESTYLE ASSESSMENT

The following questions are designed to get you thinking about aspects of your life that might be impacted by working as a doula. There are certain things that being a doula requires in order to provide your clients with support. This is a tool that can help you heighten your lifestyle-awareness while considering a career as a doula.

This questionnaire does not intend to cause self-judgment or raise concerns but often when people complete it, they start conjuring up scenarios in their minds of what their answers predict for the future. Don't worry about coming up with solutions to any complications you are imagining. Just be aware of your needs for now.

And try not to fret if you start to feel like you can't be the kind of doula you anticipated. The point of this tool is to help you be clear about your capacities so you can match your Lifestyle Assessment with the Doula Role Assessment to find the perfect doula role that will fit with your lifestyle (you'll do this using the Doula-bility Calculator).

You will learn strategies to deal with lifestyle complexities in your doula training. You can start connecting with people already working in your field. Experienced doulas are always willing to share their tricks and tips, and nurture newbies.

Work Flexibility

*Choose the **one** statement that most closely fits your current situation:*

☐ I currently work a full-time job with no flexibility	Score 0
☐ I currently work a full-time job with some flexibility	Score 1
☐ I currently work a full-time job and I can miss shifts with little to no advance notice without repercussions	Score 2
☐ I currently work a part-time job with no flexibility	Score 1
☐ I currently work a part-time job with some flexibility	Score 2
☐ I currently work a part-time job and I can miss shifts with little to no advance notice without repercussions	Score 3
☐ I currently work but have total control over my schedule	Score 4
☐ I currently don't have paid work	Score 4
Your work flexibility score:	_____

What your score means:
0-2 = Choose a doula role that allows you to schedule client work outside of your current job.
3-4 = You should have the flexibility to take clients in a doula role that requires schedule flexibility until you can quit your current job.

Step 2: Your Lifestyle Assessment

Health Flexibility	
*Choose the **one** statement that most closely fits your current situation:*	
☐ I have physical or mental health conditions that require a structured routine	Score 1
☐ I have physical conditions that prevent me from standing for long periods of time	Score 2
☐ I have physical conditions that limit my mobility (bending, squatting, walking, etc.)	Score 2
☐ I have physical conditions that limit my physical strength	Score 3
☐ I am strong and limber enough to physically support a person, stay by their side, provide continual comfort measures as needed, and stay energetically connected OR I will clearly communicate any limitations to my clients and will have a plan for how to get all of those needs met by someone other than me	Score 4
Your health flexibility score:	_____

What your score means:
1-2 = Choose a doula role that allows for scheduled meetings and no on-call work.
3 = Choose a doula role that is primarily seated work with limited physical support.
4 = Any doula role should work for you.

Diet Flexibility	
*Choose the **one** statement that most closely fits your current situation:*	
☐ I have dietary needs that require specific eating that cannot be accomodated outside my home	Score 1
☐ I have dietary needs that require specific eating that can be accomodated outside my home	Score 2
☐ I am able to get my dietary needs met with many commonly available options	Score 3
☐ I am able to eat sporadically without regular meals if necessary	Score 4
Your diet flexibility score:	_____

What your score means:
1 = Choose a doula role based on visits that are scheduled.
2-3 = Choose a doula role that allows you to bring your own meals or have access to purchasing food.
4 = You should be able to perform a doula role that is on-call and physically demanding, such as a birth doula.

Sleep Flexibility	
Choose the **one** statement that most closely fits your current situation:	
☐ I have physical or mental health conditions that require a regular sleep schedule	Score 1
☐ I have physical or mental health conditions, or medications that I must take, that prevent me from staying awake.	Score 1
☐ I am able to miss sleep ocassionally but require recovery time afterward	Score 2
☐ I am able to stay awake for long periods of time, up to 24 hours or longer, and function reasonably well.	Score 3
Your sleep flexibility score:	_____

What your score means:
1 = Choose a doula role that is based on scheduled visits.
2 = Any doula role should work for you, but limit the number of on-call clients in a given time period.
3 = On-call doula roles should work for you.

Responsibilities Flexibility	
Choose the **one** statement that most closely fits your current situation:	
☐ I have children, elders, pets, or others that I care for full-time and do not have backup care for them	Score 0
☐ I have children, elders, pets, or others that I care for part-time	Score 1
☐ I have others that give me breaks from those that I care for	Score 2
☐ I have on-call backup care for those that I care for	Score 3
☐ I do not have anyone else that I care for	Score 4
Your responsibilities flexibility score:	_____

What your score means:
0 = Choose a doula role that is schedule-based and ideally can be done from your home or virtually.
1-2 = Choose a doula role that is schedule-based.
3-4 = Any doula role should work for you.

Step 2: Your Lifestyle Assessment

Transportation Flexibility	
*Choose the **one** statement that most closely fits your current situation:*	
☐ I have reliable transportation (a car that works, bike-friendly client/birthplace locations, comprehensive public transportation, or money for rideshares/taxis)	Score 4
☐ I have access to reliable transportation	Score 3
☐ I have money to access reliable transportation	Score 2
☐ I do not have access transportation or money for transportation and must work from home	Score 1
Your transportation flexibility score:	_____

What your score means:
1 = Choose a doula role that can be done virtually from your home
2-4 = Any doula role may work for you, but be mindful of the time it takes to travel for on-call roles.

Schedule Flexibility	
*Choose the **one** statement that most closely fits your current situation:*	
☐ I am able to be on call for clients and respond to them within an hour	Score 3
☐ I am able to be on call for clients and physically join them within an hour	Score 4
☐ I am able to respond to my clients by the next day	Score 2
☐ I need a week's notice to start working with a client/add a client to my schedule	Score 1
☐ I need at least a month's lead time before working with clients on a scheduled basis	Score 0
Your schedule flexibility score:	_____

What your score means:
0 = Choose a doula role that has predictability and is schedule-based.
1-2 = Most schedule-based doula roles should work for you.
3-4 = Scheduled and on-call doula roles should work for you.

Social Life Flexibility	
*Choose the **one** statement that most closely fits your current situation:*	
☐ I have a full social life with little time for new things and I'm not willing to change it	Score 1
☐ I have a full social life with little time for new things but I'm willing to change it	Score 2
☐ I have spare time for new things in my life	Score 3
Your social life flexibility score:	_____
What your score means: 1 = Choose a doula role that is schedule-based for activities that typically occur outside your social schedule. 2-3 = Start ramping up your doula career while adjusting your social calendar	
On Call Flexibility	
*Choose the **one** statement that most closely fits your current situation:*	
☐ I have schedules or rituals that I perform at specific times that I am not able or willing to miss	Score 1
☐ I am able and willing to be on call AND my partner, family, friends, co-workers, and community understand that I am on call and may be called to a client at any time, need to cancel commitments without advance notice, and will be supportive of my work as a doula	Score 2
☐ I am able and willing to be on call AND I am willing to miss special occasions such as birthdays, holidays, graduations, and anniversaries if I'm called to fulfill my doula role.	Score 3
Your on call flexibility score:	_____
What your score means: 1 = Choose a doula role that is schedule-based and will not require working during your commitments. 2-3 = You should be able to do any doula role, including those that are on-call.	

Step 2: Your Lifestyle Assessment

Safety Flexibility	
*Choose **ALL** statements that are true for you:*	
☐ I am comfortable entering and navigating neighborhoods I haven't visited before	Score 2
☐ I am comfortable entering and navigating inside people's homes	Score 3
☐ I am not comfortable entering unfamiliar neighborhoods, places, or homes without specific directions or guidance	Score 1
☐ I am not comfortable entering unfamiliar neighborhoods, places, or homes	Score 0
☐ I am comfortable traveling and/or driving at night	Score 4
☐ I know basic personal safety and self-protection strategies.	Score 4
Your safety flexibility score:	_____

What your score means
0-3 = Choose a doula role that can be performed virtually, or occurs in a place you are familiar with or can become familiar with.
4-8 = Most doula roles should work for you.
10-15 = You are especially suited for doula roles where you could be called on at night or in isolated places.

Facilities Flexibility	
*Choose the **one** statement that most closely fits your current situation:*	
☐ I am comfortable entering and navigating medical facilities	Score 3
☐ I am comfortable entering and navigating educational facilities	Score 3
☐ I am comfortable entering and navigating in courthouses	Score 3
☐ I have worked in one of the above settings and am very comfortable there	Score 4
☐ I only enter and navigate medical facilities, schools, or courthouses when I have to	Score 1
☐ I am very uncomfortable entering and navigating in medical facilities, schools, or courthouses	Score 0
Your facilities flexibility score:	_____

What your score means:
0-1 = Choose a doula role that is based on serving people in their homes or virtually.
3-4 = A doula role in any of the settings you are comfortable in should work for you.

On Call Acknowledgment
For doula roles that require being on call (primarily birth and death doulas), read and check that you acknowledge each statement.
Birth doulas: I acknowledge that most births are not scheduled. For every client's due date, I am actually on call for 2-3 weeks before their due date and 2 weeks after their due date (a 4-6 week window). Also, clients may go into preterm labor and I would do my best to be available for them outside of that window. ☐
Death doulas: I acknowledge that most deaths are not scheduled. ☐
I understand that I must schedule vacations and other time off prior to taking clients, and that if a last-minute out-of-town opportunity comes up I will have to decline if I am on-call during that time. ☐
I will put a phone number with every entry into my calendar, in case I need to cancel if called to a client. And I will find doctors, dentists, and other professionals willing to waive their 24-hour cancellation fees for me. ☐
I will not get intoxicated any time I am on call. ☐
I will develop self-care practices that ensure I am not giving away more energy than I am restoring. ☐
I will be aware of my personal hygiene so that I am fresh and ready to go to join a client when called. ☐
I will keep my phone with me and on (vibrate if silenced) at all times that I am on call. ☐
I know other doulas to connect with for support, backup, and confidential debriefing. ☐
If I have children:
I have on-call childcare readily available at any time, any day of the week. And I have 3 levels of childcare – plan A, plan B, and plan C ☐
I have childcare that is available 24 hours a day, and that I trust to transport my child in my absence. ☐
I have childcare that will care for my children if they are sick and I get called to join a client. ☐

Step 2: Your Lifestyle Assessment

If I have a nursing child, they will accept pumped milk or other food during my absence, and I will make arrangements to express my milk while with a client.	☐
In truth, you may never experience any of these challenges, or may need to implement only a few of the strategies. Or at worst, you may only experience these hardships once in a while. But you do need to be aware of them before you enter these fields.	

Access this and all other forms online at https://doula-training.carriekenner.com/doula-assessment-forms-book

Now that you have key insights into your interests from Chapter 6 and your current lifestyle from this chapter, it's time to match them up with the doula roles that will be ideal for you.

CHAPTER 8

Step 3: Doula Role Variables

I just want to pause for a moment and say, *Congratulations!* What you have accomplished so far is extraordinary. Most people don't put this much time or thought into becoming a doula. The groundwork you are lying will be critical to your success as a doula. Well done!

In the next chapter, you're going to use the Doula-bility Calculator to match your unique *Interest Scores* from the Interest Assessment and *Flexibility Scores* from the Lifestyle Assessment to your ideal doula roles.

But first, let's take a super high-level look at doula roles through these six key variables:

- Schedulability
- Type of work
- Location
- In person or virtual
- Who you're working with
- Timeframe of the relationship

Schedulability

Schedulable Visits—Predictable Event—On-call Event

Most doula roles fall into two categories: Schedule-based or on-call. Schedule-based doula roles are those where both your individual visits with clients *and* visits you might accompany them on (to the clinic, lawyer, or funeral home) are scheduled. You may need to be available by phone or text for questions or urgent needs, but otherwise the work is quite predictable.

Next, consider whether the life event itself is scheduled (like surgery) or unpredictable (the onset of menstruation). And whether you need to be there right away or not (menstruation: no, birth: yes).

Another consideration about scheduled visits or events is how long they last. Attending court or a surgery may be multiple hours, whereas a clinical or attorney visit may take only thirty minutes (but don't forget to factor in travel time). Most individual visits with your clients are one to two hours.

On-call doula roles typically include scheduled home visits, but the part where you accompany them through the event cannot be scheduled, such as a birth or death. These events are also unpredictable in length, which is why birth and death doulas require the ultimate in flexibility.

Type of work

Sit-Down Meetings—Standing/Sitting Presence—Hands-on Physical Support

Some doula roles consist of primarily discussion-based activities. Most of the work is done via scheduled sit-down meetings either in the client's home, your office, or virtually. Physical interaction or movement is limited.

Other doula roles include hands-on support, or lots of standing and moving around. Birth, postpartum, and death doulas are prime examples of this.

Some other doula roles don't require direct physical support, but one's physical presence is a key component (fertility treatments, abortion, post gender transition surgery, weddings, pets, divorce, and psychedelic therapy specifically). Consider if the doula's presence can be done while sitting or if it needs to be standing (by the bedside, for example) to determine if a specific doula role is a good fit for you.

While some doulas may lead in-person rituals, facilitate family conversations, or coordinate multi-party discussions (such as with surrogate families or dementia care providers), much of that can be done virtually. That is a choice to be made between the doula and their clients.

Virtual or in-person

Virtual—Combo—In Person

If there is a physical hands-on component, the doula role likely needs to be done in person (though coaching a friend or loved one to provide hands-on touch may be an option, as birth doulas did during COVID).

If the doula role includes accompanying a client to a meeting or visit, through an event, or to lead a ritual or activity, it is usually done in person (though, again, virtual attendance is possible but often not as effective).

If the doula role is primarily discussion-based or verbal support for events that are scheduled or predictable, does not require physical support or hands-on comfort, and skills or exercises can be demonstrated or self-guided, then virtual sessions are a great option.

Many doulas have clients worldwide and do all their work remotely. Even though doulas and clients may never meet in person, they form a wonderful bond.

Location

Home/Office—Facility

The location refers to where the life event is happening. Most doula roles will include a combination of private visits with clients in their homes, your office, or virtually, and possibly accompanying clients when they visit other professionals.

For most of the medically-related doula roles (cancer and illness, infertility or abortion), the main event will happen in a clinic or hospital. Some medical events can also happen at home, such as birth, death, or miscarriage.

Doula roles having to do with legal issues—such as divorce, court, or incarceration—will happen in the judicial system in a courthouse.

Then there are situation-specific locations, such as a veterinary office for pets, or a wedding site for marriage.

Who you're working with

Individual—Couple/Family—Professionals in the Field

Doulas typically work with an individual or an individual and their family. Divorce doulas almost always work with just their client. Doulas working in the childbearing field are usually working with a couple. When a doula works with more than one person, they rarely meet with any one person individually, as a way to keep the relationships balanced and unbiased.

Most doulas work primarily with adults. They may be involved in the care of infants or children, or children might be a part of the family they are working with, but the primary relationship is with the parents.

Doulas working with medical events will often be interacting with medical professionals such as doctors, nurses, and technicians. Doulas working in the judicial field will have interactions with lawyers, judges, and court clerks. I don't want to mislead you to think doulas are having direct or private conversations with these folks in lieu of their clients, but they may be present when their clients are meeting with them.

Doulas may also be in the presence of industry-specific professionals such as veterinarians, wedding planners, adoption agencies, psychedelic therapists, or funeral directors.

Timeframe of the relationship

Weeks—Months—Years

A doula's relationship with their clients may last a few weeks or years, depending on the life transition. Menopause doulas may provide support for years throughout perimenopause and menopause. Pet adoption doulas may work with a family for a week or two.

Most doulas start working with a family soon after they learn of an upcoming life transition (a medical diagnosis, pregnancy, gender transition, engagement, separation, or loss) and support them until a few weeks or months after the event has occurred. The length of the relationship depends on the duration of the situation.

How a doula and client work together during the duration may vary greatly. There may be many meetings for discussing, learning, and planning at first, followed by periodic check-in visits or attending appointments, followed by a few follow-up visits. Or there may be regular meetings scheduled throughout the relationship.

Most doulas will let clients know how long to expect working together, and they may mutually decide when it is time to end the relationship.

How do the doula roles measure up?

Reproduction Doulas

Menstruation

- Schedulability: *schedulable visits*
- The type of work: *sit-down meetings*
- Virtual or in person: *virtual, in person, or both*
- Location: *home/office*
- Who you're working with: *individual*
- Timeframe of the relationship: *months*

Birth Control

- Schedulability: *schedulable visits*
- The type of work: *sit-down meetings*
- Virtual or in person: *virtual, in person, or both*
- Location: *home/office*
- Who you're working with: *individual*
- Timeframe of the relationship: *months*

Preconception

- Schedulability: *schedulable visits*
- The type of work: *sit-down meetings*
- Virtual or in person: *virtual, in person, or both*
- Location: *home/office*
- Who you're working with: *couples or individuals*
- Timeframe of the relationship: *months*

Fertility/Infertility

- Schedulability: *schedulable visits*
- The type of work: *sit-down meetings*
- Virtual or in person: *virtual, in person, or both*
- Location: *home/office and facility*
- Who you're working with: *couples, professionals in the field*
- Timeframe of the relationship: *months to years*

Abortion

- Schedulability: *schedulable visits and predictable event*
- The type of work: *sit-down meetings, standing or sitting presence, active hands-on physical support*
- Virtual or in person: *virtual and in person*
- Location: *home/office and medical facility*
- Who you're working with: *couples or individual*
- Timeframe of the relationship: *weeks*

Miscarriage

- Schedulability: *on-call event*
- The type of work: *standing or sitting presence, active hands-on physical support*
- Virtual or in person: *virtual and in person*
- Location: *home/office and medical facility*
- Who you're working with: *individual, couple, and professionals in the field*
- Timeframe of the relationship: *weeks*

Surrogacy

- Schedulability: *schedulable visits and on-call event*
- The type of work: *sit-down meetings, standing or sitting presence, active hands-on physical support*

- Virtual or in person: *virtual and in person*
- Location: *home/office and medical facility*
- Who you're working with: *individual and/or couple and professionals in the field*
- Timeframe of the relationship: *months*

Antepartum/Antenatal (aka Bed Rest)

- Schedulability: *schedulable visits*
- The type of work: *sit-down meetings, standing or sitting presence, active hands-on physical support*
- Virtual or in person: *virtual and in person*
- Location: *home/office and medical facility*
- Who you're working with: *individual or couple/family and professionals in the field*
- Timeframe of the relationship: *weeks to months*

Birth

- Schedulability: *schedulable visits and on-call event*
- The type of work: *sit-down meetings, standing or sitting presence, active hands-on physical support*
- Virtual or in person: *virtual and in person*
- Location: *home/office and medical facility*
- Who you're working with: *individual or couple/family and professionals in the field*
- Timeframe of the relationship: *months*

Postpartum

- Schedulability: *schedulable visits*
- The type of work: *standing or sitting presence, active hands-on physical support*
- Virtual or in person: *virtual and in person*
- Location: *home/office*

- Who you're working with: *individual or couple/family*
- Timeframe of the relationship: *weeks to months*

Life Transition Doulas

Menarche

- Schedulability: *schedulable visits*
- The type of work: *sit-down meetings*
- Virtual or in-person: *virtual, in-person, or both*
- Location: *home/office*
- Who you're working with: *individual*
- Timeframe of the relationship: *weeks*

Gender and/or Gender Transition

- Schedulability: *schedulable visits, predictable event*
- The type of work: *sit-down meetings, standing or sitting presence*
- Virtual or in person: *virtual, in person, or both*
- Location: *home/office and medical facility*
- Who you're working with: *individual or family and professionals in the field*
- Timeframe of the relationship: *weeks to months*

Marriage and/or Wedding

- Schedulability: *schedulable visits, predictable event*
- The type of work: *sit-down meetings, standing or sitting presence*
- Virtual or in person: *virtual, in person, or both*
- Location: *home/office and wedding facility*
- Who you're working with: *couple, maybe family and professionals in the field*
- Timeframe of the relationship: *months*

Adoption

- Schedulability: *schedulable visits*
- The type of work: *sit-down meetings*
- Virtual or in person: *virtual, in person, or both*
- Location: *home/office*
- Who you're working with: *individual or couple/family and professionals in the field*
- Timeframe of the relationship: *months*

Pet Adoption or Loss

- Schedulability: *schedulable visits*
- The type of work: *sit-down meetings*
- Virtual or in person: *virtual, in-person, or both*
- Location: *home/office*
- Who you're working with: *individual or family*
- Timeframe of the relationship: *weeks*

Menopause

- Schedulability: *schedulable visits*
- The type of work: *sit-down meetings*
- Virtual or in person: *virtual, in person, or both*
- Location: *home/office*
- Who you're working with: *individual*
- Timeframe of the relationship: *months to years*

Divorce

- Schedulability: *schedulable visits, predictable event*
- The type of work: *sit-down meetings, standing or sitting presence*
- Virtual or in person: *virtual, in person, or both*
- Location: *home/office and courts*
- Who you're working with: *individual and professionals in the field*

- Timeframe of the relationship: *months*

Court or Judicial System

- Schedulability: *schedulable visits, predictable event*
- The type of work: *sit-down meetings, standing or sitting presence*
- Virtual or in person: *virtual, in person, or both*
- Location: *home/office and courts*
- Who you're working with: *individual or family and professionals in the field*
- Timeframe of the relationship: *months*

Incarceration

- Schedulability: *schedulable visits*
- The type of work: *sit-down meetings*
- Virtual or in person: *virtual, in person, or both*
- Location: *home/office, maybe courts*
- Who you're working with: *individual or family*
- Timeframe of the relationship: *weeks or months*

Grief

- Schedulability: *schedulable visits*
- The type of work: *sit-down meetings*
- Virtual or in person: *virtual, in person, or both*
- Location: *home/office*
- Who you're working with: *individual or family*
- Timeframe of the relationship: *weeks to months*

Dementia

- Schedulability: *schedulable visits*
- The type of work: *sit-down meetings*
- Virtual or in person: *virtual, in person, or both*

- Location: *home/office*
- Who you're working with: *individual or family*
- Timeframe of the relationship: *months to years*

End of Life

- Schedulability: *schedulable visits*
- The type of work: *sit-down meetings, standing or sitting presence*
- Virtual or in person: *virtual, in person, or both*
- Location: *home/office*
- Who you're working with: *individual or family and professionals in the field*
- Timeframe of the relationship: *weeks to months*

Death

- Schedulability: *schedulable visits, on-call event*
- The type of work: *sit-down meetings, standing or sitting presence, active hands-on physical support*
- Virtual or in person: *virtual and in person*
- Location: *home/office, maybe funeral facility*
- Who you're working with: *individual or family and professionals in the field*
- Timeframe of the relationship: *weeks to months*

Medical Doulas

Cancer

- Schedulability: *schedulable visits*
- The type of work: *sit-down meetings, standing or sitting presence, active hands-on physical support*
- Virtual or in person: *virtual and in person*
- Location: *home/office and medical facility*

- Who you're working with: *individual and/or family and professionals in the field*
- Timeframe of the relationship: *months*

Illness

- Schedulability: *schedulable visits*
- The type of work: *sit-down meetings, standing or sitting presence*
- Virtual or in person: *virtual and in person*
- Location: *home/office and medical facility*
- Who you're working with: *individual and/or family and professionals in the field*
- Timeframe of the relationship: *weeks or months*

Psychedelic Therapy

- Schedulability: *schedulable visits, predictable event*
- The type of work: *sit-down meetings, standing or sitting presence*
- Virtual or in person: *virtual and in person*
- Location: *home/office and therapy facility*
- Who you're working with: *individual and professionals in the field*
- Timeframe of the relationship: *weeks to months*

CHAPTER 9

Step 4: The Doula-bility Calculator

Yay! Finally, we get to put it all together. Are you ready to find out what doula roles would be a good fit for you? I bet you already have a good idea from reading the past eight chapters. Let's see how it all shakes out in The Doula-bility Calculator!

You'll be using your Interest Scores from the Interest Assessment and Flexibility Scores from the Lifestyle Assessment, so have them handy.

SO YOU WANT TO BE A DOULA

LIFESTYLE SECTION		REPRODUCTION DOULAS								
		Menstruation	Birth Control	Preconception	Fertility/Infertility	Abortion	Miscarriage	Surrogacy	Antepartum/Antenatal	Birth	Postpartum
FLEXIBILITY SCORES											
1. Enter your Flexibility Scores from the Lifestyle Assessment in this column: ⬇											
Work Flexibility		All	All	All	2-3	4	4	3-4	2-3	4	3-4
Health Flexibility		All	All	All	All	3-4	3-4	3-4	3-4	3-4	3-4
Diet Flexibility		All	All	All	All	3-4	3-4	3-4	2-4	3-4	2-4
Sleep Flexilibity		All	All	All	All	2-3	2-3	2-3	All	2-3	2-3
Responsibilities Flexibility		All	All	All	All	3-4	3-4	3-4	1-4	3-4	1-4
Transportation Flexibility		All	All	All	2-4	2-4	2-4	2-4	2-4	2-4	2-4
Schedule Flexibility		All	All	All	1-4	3-4	3-4	3-4	1-4	3-4	1-4
Social Life Flexibility		All	All	All	All	3	3	2-3	2-3	3	2-3
On-call Flexibility		All	All	All	All	3	3	3	All	3	All
Safety Flexibility		All	All	All	All	10-15	All	4-15	4-15	10-15	4-15
Facilities Flexibility		All	All	All	3-4	3-4	3-4	3-4	3-4	3-4	3-4
2. Circle every cell above that has one of your scores in it.											
3. Then, put an X in this row for every doula role column that would fit with your lifestyle ➡											

Step 4: The Doula-bility Calculator

Life Transition Doulas													Medical Doulas		
Menarche	Gender Transition	Marriage and/or Wedding	Adoption	Pet adoption or loss	Menopause	Divorce	Court or Judicial System	Incarceration	Grief	Dementia	End of Life	Death	Cancer	Illness	Psychedelic therapy
All	2-4	All	2-4	3-4	All	2-4	2-4	2-4	All	2-4	2-4	4	2-4	2-4	All
All	2-4	2-4	All	All	All	All	All	All	All	All	3-4	3-4	2-4	All	All
All	2-4	2-4	All	All	All	3-4	3-4	3-4	All	2-4	3-4	3-4	3-4	2-4	3-4
All	All	All	All	All	All	All	All	All	All	All	2-3	2-3	All	All	All
All	1-4	1-4	1-4	1-4	All	1-4	1-4	1-4	All	1-4	3-4	3-4	1-4	1-4	1-4
All	2-4	2-4	2-4	2-4	All	2-4	2-4	2-4	All	2-4	2-4	2-4	2-4	2-4	2-4
All	1-4	1-4	1-4	2-4	All	2-4	2-4	2-4	2-4	2-4	3-4	3-4	1-4	1-4	All
All	2-3	3	2-3	2-3	All	2-3	2-3	2-3	2-3	2-3	3	3	2-3	2-3	All
All	All	All	All	All	All	All	All	All	All	All	3	3	All	All	All
All	4-15	4-15	All	All	All	4-15	4-15	4-15	All	All	10-15	10-15	4-15	4-15	All
All	3-4	3-4	All	All	All	3-4	3-4	3-4	All	All	3-4	3-4	3-4	3-4	1-4

SO YOU WANT TO BE A DOULA

INTERESTS SECTION		REPRODUCTION DOULAS									
		Menstruation	Birth Control	Preconception	Fertility/Infertility	Abortion	Miscarriage	Surrogacy	Antepartum	Birth	Postpartum
AREAS OF INTEREST											
1. Enter your Codes from the Interest Assessment in this column: ⬇											
Gender		All	All	All	All	W,G	W,G	All	W,G	W,G	All
Medical		W,G	X	W,M,G	W,M,G	W,G	W,G	W,M,G	W,G	W,G	W,M,G
Age		T,L	T,L	L	L	T,L	T,L	L	T,L	T,L	T,L
Reproduction		R	BD	F	F	A	MC	SR	PB	PB	PP
Life Transitions		T,G	T,G	n/a	n/a	GR	GR	GR	n/a	PA	PA
2. Circle every cell above that has one of your codes in it.											
3. Then, put an X in this row for every doula role column that has 3 or more circles in it ➡											

Step 4: The Doula-bility Calculator

LIFE TRANSITION DOULAS													MEDICAL DOULAS		
Menarche	Gender and/or Gender Transition	Marriage and/or Wedding	Adoption	Pet adoption or loss	Menopause	Divorce	Court or Judicial System	Incarceration	Grief	Dementia	End of Life	Death	Cancer	Illness	Psychedelic therapy
W,G	G	All	All	n/a	W,G	All	n/a	n/a	n/a	n/a	n/a	n/a	n/a	n/a	n/a
W,G	G, S	n/a	n/a	n/a	W,G	n/a	n/a	n/a	n/a	E	D,E	D,E	CA	IL	PS
T	All	L	L	n/a	MP	L	All	All	All	L,E	All	All	All	All	L,E
R	F,PB	F	n/a	n/a	R	n/a	n/a	n/a	n/a	n/a	n/a	n/a	n/a	n/a	n/a
T	G	MR	O,PA	P	MP	DV	C	I	GR	E	D	D	GR	GR	D

SO YOU WANT TO BE A DOULA

DOULA ROLE VARIABLES SECTION		REPRODUCTION DOULAS									
		Menstruation	Birth Control	Preconception	Fertility/Infertility	Abortion	Miscarriage	Surrogacy	Antepartum	Birth	Postpartum
1. Now, put an X under every doula role that has an X from BOTH the Lifestyle and Interest sections above: ➡											
2. Put an X for every doula role variables you desire in this column: ⬇		➡ 3. Then, put a big X in every cell below									
Schedulability											
Schedulable											
Predictable											
On call											
Type of work											
Sit down											
Standing or Sitting											
Hands-on Phys. Support											
Format											
Virtual											
Combo											
In Person											
Locations											
Home/Office											
Facility											

Step 4: The Doula-bility Calculator

	LIFE TRANSITION DOULAS											MEDICAL DOULAS		
Menarche	Gender and/or Gender Transition	Marriage and/or Wedding	Adoption	Pet adoption or loss	Menopause	Divorce	Court or Judicial System	Incarceration	Grief	Dementia	End of Life	Death	Cancer	Illness	Psychedelic therapy

that has an X in the top row and an X in the left column.

97

SO YOU WANT TO BE A DOULA

DOULA ROLE VARIABLES SECTION (cont'd.)		Menstruation	Birth Control	Preconception	Fertility/Infertility	Abortion	Miscarriage	Surrogacy	Antepartum	Birth	Postpartum
		\multicolumn{11}{c	}{REPRODUCTION DOULAS}
1. Again, put an X under every doula role that has an X from BOTH the Lifestyle and Interest sections above: ➡											
2. Put an X for every doula role variables you desire in this column: ⬇		➡ 3. Then, put a big X in every cell below									
Working With											
Individual											
Couple/Family											
Professionals in the field											
Length of Relationship											
Weeks											
Months											
Years											
4. Finally, put an X in this row for the 3-4 columns in the Doula Role Variables section that have the most circles ➡											

You should now be able to see which doula roles match with your lifestyle,

Step 4: The Doula-bility Calculator

	LIFE TRANSITION DOULAS										MEDICAL DOULAS		
Menarche	Gender and/or Gender Transition	Marriage and/or Wedding	Adoption	Pet adoption or loss	Menopause	Divorce	Court or Judicial System	Incarceration	Grief	Dementia	End of Life	Death	Cancer	Illness	Psychedelic therapy

that has an X in the top row and an X in the left column.

interests, and variables of the role. Congratulations, you've met your match(es)!

Access this and all other forms online at https://doula-training.carriekenner.com/doula-assessment-forms-book

Now that you've completed the Doula-bility Calculator you should have a few doulas roles that you know will fit your lifestyle, interests, and doula role attributes. So, now what?

Well, one of three things may have happened:

1. You aren't surprised at all by the results. You've known all along what your ideal role would be and it was confirmed here.
2. You got some great insights and options. All you have to do is choose!
3. It's not at all what you expected. A few of the roles you matched with you'd never considered before, and a few that you were really interested in would not be a good match. You have some thinking to do.

If you fall into the first category, yay! Just keep reading the next chapters to continue your doula career.

If you're in the second category, you might take some time to think about your options. Talk with people who know you well and ask for their insights to provide perspective. If you're really having a hard time choosing between multiple options, I suggest you create a two- to five-year plan for expanding your doula practice. Start with one doula role (the easiest one, perhaps), then add a second or third one down the road.

If you're in category number three, you have a few options. What you decide to do next will depend on how much flexibility you have in your life right now. If you have some flexibility, take a look at what specific things you'd need to address to match with a role you were really interested in. Do you have to be more comfortable in public facilities? Or do you need to open up your schedule for doula clients? If you can act on any of these specific changes, come up with a plan to make those adjustments and proceed with your doula training.

If you don't have the capacity for much change in your current life, are you interested in one of the "surprise" roles you matched with? This might be an easy way to get your feet wet as a doula and start practicing the foundational skills. Who knows, you might love this unexpected role and stick with it! Or, it might provide the springboard you need and create more space in your life to pursue the doula role your heart desires. Either way, you'll be on the road to becoming a doula and gaining experience.

> **Key Chapter Takeaways**
>
> There are seven major questions that all doulas must answer for themselves before they start the training process. The Interest Assessment, Lifestyle Assessment, and Doula-ability Calculator help you answer all those questions:
>
> 1. Why am I interested in this particular doula role?
> 2. Will my lifestyle fit with this role?
> 3. Am I financially ready to make the leap to doula work?
> 4. What kind of lifestyle adjustments might be required to become a doula—and am I able and willing to make them?
> 5. What obstacles might discourage or prevent me from pursuing this role?
> 6. Will I feel safe in this role?
> 7. What similar roles might be a better or similar fit?

CHAPTER 10

What Does It Take to Be a Doula?

In Chapter 3, I discussed the key principles and primary skills for all doulas. Now, let's look at additional qualities that doulas bring to their work.

Passion

The desire to be a doula is typically born of a combination of past experience and hearing about this new role. There is something in the heart of every doula that tugged, flickered, or burned to be felt and seen. Something that pulled you down a specific aisle in the library, turned your head every time you saw a potential client, or kept you up for hours watching YouTube videos on your topic of interest. There is something deep inside you that drew you to this work.

You could have channeled your interests into technical, clinical, or policy roles. But at some point, you heard about doulas and the light bulb clicked on: *This is it, this is what I want to do!* A wise voice inside of you discerned how a doula differs from those other roles, and a wise listener then heard the call.

The doula role combines being with people in times of stress, working intimately with individuals and their families, and being of service. It protects you from years of education and school loans that may never get used. It frees you (somewhat) from blood and guts and life and death responsibility.

The doula role is like no other. You can learn how to be a doula in a few days, weeks, or months and start practicing right away. In fact, you may have already done it without any training, and I bet you were great!

The "Soft" Skills

The best mentors and guides are people who have done their own inner work first. I designed the *Becoming a Doula Journal* to help guide doulas through their own inner journey as they become a doula, and I encourage you to use this journal to aid in your personal exploration.

As a doula, you may be guiding people through one of the most transformational times of their life. I learned this approach to birth support in my training with Pam England, MSW, CNM, based on her seminal book *Birthing From Within*. I worked for twenty years as a Birthing From Within mentor, advisor, facilitator, and co-owner. What Birthing From Within taught me was this:

To truly be with another person, to be in the moment with them, to sit at the edge of the unknown, **you must explore your inner terrain***, and then you can guide others through theirs.*

Here's what you need to know to do that:

Your primary role as a doula is that of mentor.

men·tor

/ˈmenˌtôr,ˈmenˌtər/

noun

noun: **mentor**; plural noun: **mentors**

1. an experienced and trusted adviser.

Mentors are not experts, but they know something of the path ahead. Mentors ask lots of questions and listen deeply to learn where their clients are coming from. They meet them where they are at. They believe that their clients already have the answers within, and they help clients to excavate their own inner knowing.

Mentors accompany clients along their unique journey, rather than lead them. From this client-centered role, you will escort clients through their own internal exploration, help them prepare for the upcoming event, and walk alongside them through whatever situations arise.

As a doula, you should experience and practice every tool and skill you use to prepare your clients for what lies ahead. You should answer for yourself all the questions you ask them. This is what builds the insight, empathy, and humility that is essential to doula work. Mentors are often described as folks who hold up a mirror to others. You need to have taken a good long look in the mirror before you can hold it up to your clients.

A doula who has done their own inner exploration is compassionate and non-judgmental. You will help clients explore their beliefs and values, which will influence the choices they make. You will help them make preparations and navigate the emotional and physical terrain of the various systems they encounter. You will encourage them to ask questions and access resources throughout their experience.

A doula accompanies and witnesses their client's ordeal, provides emotional and physical support along the way, and helps them integrate their experience during the return (the concepts of the ordeal and return are part of the heroic journey that is explored in the *Becoming a Doula Journal*).

When this type of comprehensive and soulful support is provided, clients are more prepared for the unknown, less traumatized by the twists and turns of life-altering events, less dogmatic, and more open to the gifts their journey will bring. When challenges are approached in this way, people are able to more readily experience their situation as a transformation, and integrate what they learn as they evolve into their new roles.

P.S. You are absolutely NOT required to have been through what your clients are facing in order to be a great doula. When I talk about "experience" and "having walked the path," I am referring to one's experience with doing inner work: introspection, reflection, and initiation. Knowledge of the process, familiarity with the related systems, and the intersections of racism, social justice, and marginalization is the basic body of knowledge of the doula role.

> You know that feeling when you don't know something yet, but you know there is something you are supposed to learn? That is the intuition that comes before learning. A wise doula knows they have to scrutinize their own ideas before they can guide someone else through theirs.
>
> Just as your clients will learn gifts from their experience that they will take into the future, you will learn gifts from becoming a doula that you will take into your family and community. You will grow exponentially from being a doula.
>
> Exploring within will help you understand a deeper meaning of what it is to be a doula, what it is to serve, and what drew you to this work. To track your growth and explore the meaning of doing this work, the *Becoming a Doula Journal* is a great accompaniment to this book.

Communication Skills: The Doula's Superpower

Communication is absolutely the most important skill you will need as a doula. Most people come to doula work thinking their job is to know enough technical information to answer questions and educate their clients. Maybe they want to throw in some hands-on techniques for physical support and have a list of resources and they're good to go.

But the doula role requires so much more! Doulas must be exquisite listeners, and learn many nuanced communication skills. In my experience as a doula trainer, communication is the topic that most doulas are surprised by, the skills they are most challenged with, and the part of their training that they are most grateful for.

"To listen another's soul into a condition of disclosure and discovery may be almost the greatest service one human being ever performs for another."
— Douglas Steere, Quaker author

You've known since you were an infant—before you learned the meaning of words and before you learned how to talk—how to read facial expressions, feel energy, hear inflections in voices, observe body positions, and mirror those around you. These innate, pre-language forms of communication form the basis of the communication skills that you will use as a doula.

Unfortunately, much of your innate knowledge of how to communicate has been "turned off." As you grew up, you were conditioned to focus just on the words, which only engage the left side of your brain. Why is this a problem?

The left side of your brain processes things in a linear way, taking the words literally and organizing them into concise thoughts. And why is that a problem?

Because people tend to say (or "put into words") only what they think they are *supposed* to think or feel or say, and a whole lot of other stuff gets censored. A good doula knows how to listen beyond the words for the buried treasure!

The good news is that you DO have instinctive skills for unspoken communication that are still intact, even if they have been overshadowed by words.

Fifty-five percent of human communication is non-verbal, such as head movements, facial expressions, body stance, eye movements, and gestures. That means the majority of "content" in communication is non-verbal.

You can tap into those instinctive ways when talking to another person by using all your senses to communicate.

What do your eyes see?

Facial expressions: What are their eyes saying? Where are they looking? What is their facial expression? Is their expression congruent with their words?

Body language: Where are their arms? Is their chest or torso open or covered? Are they rigid or soft? Are they upright or shrinking right before your eyes?

What do your ears hear?

Tone of voice or inflection: Do they sound certain? Questioning? Timid? Doubtful? Angry? Excited? Fearful?

Silence: What isn't being said? What is between the lines of the spoken words?

What do your heart and gut feel?

Intuition: What does your "gut" feel, hear, or think about what they are saying? Do you believe it? Do you think there's something more? Or do you think they are hiding something?

Energy: Soften your own energy, especially around your heart, so you can connect with their energy. What do you tap into—without thinking, but *feeling*—with them?

Now that you've awakened your innate ways of being in communication, let's move on to some technical skills you can learn.

The majority of communicating you will be doing with clients involves listening. You may have heard of "active listening" or "attentive listening." If you are familiar with them, you are well on your way to being a great listener. If not, here are some ideas.

> ### Seven Ways to Become a Better Listener
>
> 1. Listen more than you speak.
>
> 2. If random thoughts come up, let them go and bring your thoughts back to your client.
>
> 3. Stop yourself when you have the impulse to interrupt. Take a big breath and let the impulse pass.
>
> 4. If you find yourself thinking about what you will say when it is "your turn" to speak, you are no longer listening. Give your unconditional attention until your client has said what they need to say. Trust that the right words will come to you when it's your turn to speak.
>
> 5. Listening is not just about hearing with your ears. It also involves "listening" with your eyes (noticing body language), with your heart (hearing the emotion and listening with an open heart and compassion), and with your belly/gut (noticing what "rings true"—or not—or what isn't being said). Learn to recognize red flags!
>
> 6. Look at the person who is speaking. Think about what they are saying or asking. Listen for the "music behind the words."
>
> 7. Confirm what you think you've heard by clarifying, paraphrasing, or reflecting what you believe is the gist of what your client is saying. Check in with them. This will allow them to clarify if you've misunderstood, to elaborate if there is more understanding needed, and perhaps for them to "hear" their own words for the first time.

Now that you know how to listen, create a good set of questions to get your clients talking. In your doula training, you may learn a basic list of topics and questions that all clients should be asked. But knowing how to "riff" with questions is the hallmark of a skilled doula.

The most reliable questions we use as doulas are called "open-ended questions." These are questions that cannot be answered with a few words, like with a "yes" or "no," or with a trite answer like "fine," "sure," or "nah" (those answers are for "closed-ended questions"). Open-ended questions can be used in any conversation to help your client dig deeper, and to enhance your listening abilities. Here are some examples of open-ended questions:

- Tell me what you've heard/read about that.
- Tell me more… (about whatever they've just said)
- Can you say more about that? I want to make sure I understand.
- What is it like for you to hear/know that now?
- What was that like for you (when it happened)?
- How do you feel/what do you think about that experience now?
- What did you learn from that experience?

These questions are what I call "soft commands." They should not feel threatening or demanding, and yet your client feels compelled to answer. Not because you are scary and forcing them to, but because you are kind and interested and they can tell you care. So they are willing to go deeper with you.

It's important to note that this isn't how we typically engage in conversations with people, especially people who are still relative strangers! You have to ease into this type of conversation by conducting a bit of small talk, maybe handling some official business, and sharing a bit about how each other's day was. Also, don't rush the conversations. Doulas use silence a lot to indicate that they aren't in a hurry, that they are patient and willing to listen, and that what their client has to say is important and worth the wait.

Most people are not accustomed to sitting in silence and contemplation. It's a difficult thing for most Westerners to deal with. We are conditioned to fill our space with sound, noise, music, ANYthing to avoid being alone with our thoughts. And doulas are no exception.

It can also be uncomfortable for clients to have the conversational spotlight shining solely on them. Let your question sink in, allow their brain to process the question, let them observe the thoughts and emotions that come up for them and decide if it's safe to share. You MUST allow time for that to happen. Which means YOU must be patient and silent.

When I was starting out as a doula, I would ask my client an open-ended question and then silently count to ten in my head: one... two... three... four... five... six... seven... eight... Usually, by the time I got to nine, they would start answering. If I wasn't patient (or more likely, if I was nervous about the silence), I would have moved on to something else and "let them off the hook," not waiting for their thoughts to bubble to the surface, not allowing the space for deep sharing to occur.

Getting used to sitting in silence, and patiently waiting, may be one of your biggest challenges. But these open-ended questions, and the silence that follows, are the fertile ground that your doula relationship will grow in.

Practice this skill with friends and family. They will think you are behaving strangely; you will probably feel pretty weird. But do it anyway. Please trust me on this, and see what happens.

What Next?

When you ask an open-ended question and they answer, the first thing you want to do is validate what they say. As they are sharing with you, feel into what they are saying. Use the "Seven Ways to Become a Better Listener" above to help you listen deeply.

Validation is not about agreeing with them, or judging them, or "cheerleading" them. Validation is empathy, feeling into their experience, and letting them know you hear them, such as:

"That sounds like it was really painful"
"It sounds like you really care about what your mom thinks."
"Wow, you had to work really hard to get through that."
"I really hear the pride in your voice when you talk about that time."

Once your client feels well-listened to and "heard" (i.e. validated), they will feel safe to continue if there is more to say. If you rush into the next question that you've been planning in your mind (in other words, not really listening), your client may not feel that their disclosure was received, that their experience was honored, or that you care. And they will not respond to further questions as openly.

You can also paraphrase—repeat back to them what you heard them say—to make sure you understand them correctly. Paraphrasing also signals that you are truly listening to them, and reinforces that they can trust you.

Consider yourself an honored guest in the home of their lived experience; treat it as a privilege, and behave accordingly. That is the role of the doula as listener.

"Hard" Skills

If you will be working in healthcare-related fields, you may be learning some specific hands-on skills. You might learn how to do a hand massage, how to take a blood pressure, ways to hold and soothe a baby, how to change a surgical bandage, or how to calm a dementia client.

You might learn specific ways for adoptive parents to prepare their home. How to fill out legal forms. How to lead a grief ritual. How to wash a dead body

You will learn the skills necessary for your field in your doula training. And most doulas will take additional training to learn more hands-on skills from other branches of care that may apply to their field (massage, acupuncture, energy work, aromatherapy, etc.).

Technical Information

Information is not a skill, but it's a key part of what it takes to be a doula. Much of the technical information you'll need for your doula role will be learned in your particular doula training. You will also learn from books, videos, consulting with others in the field, and most of all, from experience on the job.

If you already work in the field in which you'll be a doula, you probably have this part done already. Yay!

If you are entering a new field, get ready to devour a bunch of information. Don't worry, there are rarely tests. You aren't expected to know everything before you begin working. And you can get information in many forms to match your learning style (more about that in the next chapter).

For now, just remember that technical information is a fraction of your doula role. And that this is one job where you get to choose where you specialize, based on your personal interests. A perfect match!

Practice

We all know how to get good at new skills: practice!

One of the best things about becoming a doula is that you usually don't have to start being one to lots of clients immediately. You have plenty of time to practice!

Enlist your family and friends to help you develop your intuitive skills, try out new communication styles, practice your hands-on skills, and conduct information sessions.

And always, always continue evolving as an individual.

Part 3

Find the Training That's Right for You

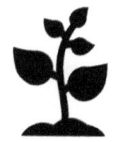

Here's a common scenario that happens after someone decides they want to become a doula:

Poised in front of a glowing screen, the aspiring doula bounces from website to website trying to devour all the information they can about becoming a doula and choose a doula training to begin right away. After all, they are excited and eager to get started.

One training they find is all online and they can start any time, but they'd really like someone live to talk to once in a while. Another training is live and virtual...but started last month, so cross that off the list. Here's one that starts this month, but it's a nine-month program and they don't want the training to take that long. Ooh, here's an in-person training in the next state over in two months...but it's $2,000!

They're off to a rocky start. So our aspiring doula turns to social media. They look for a few doula groups and find many. They choose the one that has the most followers. Okay, back on track!

They introduce themselves and post the following innocent question: "Hey doulas. Do you have any recommendations for a postpartum doula training? I'd like to start soon. I don't care if it's online or in person, but I'd like some human contact and don't want it to take more than a few months. I can afford up to $800."

They wait...and the following morning they've received 114 comments! Woah. Every commenter says the one they took is best (well, except a few who bash a program here and there). It's like a doula-training pissing contest. If a member likes a training mentioned in a comment, they comment on the comment and the original commenter likes their comment and they agree to meet up on DMs and they've posted six times on the thread about their new connection.

Meanwhile, our aspiring doula checks out a few of the trainings that many members recommended, but it feels like the members didn't read the criteria at all! There are nine-month and twelve-month options, many cost over one thousand dollars, and some aren't even for postpartum doulas.

Exasperated, they look at a few of the doulas who provided thoughtful responses and reach out to them personally. Those doulas give some guidance of what to look for and suggest how to navigate their choices, and our aspiring doula decides on one that looks good enough. They cross their fingers, enter their credit card number, and hit [ENROLL].

Why is this awful scenario so common? Because there are so many choices and no guidance on how to go through the options in a systematic way.

Until now.

It's not about your resources, it's about your resourcefulness.

It's not any aspiring doula's fault that it's so hard to find the right doula training for them. When a potential doula is looking for recommendations, they're asking doulas who have typically taken only one training. Can those doulas really say if theirs was better or not? And most doula trainers don't differentiate their training from others. In fact, most doula trainings sound a lot alike.

But there are many differences in training philosophies, delivery method, content, and style that could help the savvy shopper.

So, if you've experienced this, it's not your fault. Let's get on track to finding a great doula training for *you*.

After you complete the assessments in Part 3, you'll know which doula training you want to take and the steps to start your training journey.

CHAPTER 11

Your Learning Style(s)

How do you prefer to learn? Do you like to read an instruction manual, watch a demo on YouTube, listen to someone explain it to you, or figure it out by doing it yourself? Maybe you need a combination of two of those to learn best.

We all have preferences for how we like to learn. But we also have to be honest about if we really learn best that way. We rarely use just one way to learn, so consider this...

You may *like* to listen to podcasts to learn information but can you recall what was said?

You may watch many video tutorials but do you retain the concepts in addition to the images in your mind?

You may read a textbook but can you apply the information in the real world?

All of these are examples of how we take in information, but we always need to be aware if we are *learning* it.

Learning is the process of acquiring new understanding, knowledge, behaviors, skills, values, attitudes, and preferences.

It's something we do every day, without noticing it much of the time, and our minds and bodies are hard-wired to do it. And as we were reminded in the previous chapter, we need to practice what we're learning to do it well.

The concept of *learning styles* (as the one way we learn best) has been debated by psychologists, educators, and scientists for decades. While most people do have a *preference* (what they enjoy most or perceive to be most effective), nobody learns in only one way. Our brains are too complex for that type of simplicity.

The human brain is built to receive information via all its senses—visual, auditory, felt, taste, smell, equilibrioception, proprioception, chronoception, and intuition. All senses are required for our survival and using all of them strengthens the synaptic connections in our bodies.

Since our brains and bodies are hardwired for all these senses, teaching approaches that use all of them is beneficial.

In addition to *how* information is shared, there are a gazillion variables that affect *how* well we learn it, such as the quality of an instructor, their choice of words and phrases, teaching tools (visual aids, demonstrations, examples, exercises), and our surroundings. Heck, even our mood at any given moment affects how well we learn.

All that being said, it can be helpful to identify how we prefer to take in information and what distracts us from learning. Having insights like this about ourselves can be helpful as long as we don't view those insights as limiting.

There is an assessment you can do that helps you identify if you *prefer* certain learning styles—visual (V), auditory (A) or kinesthetic (K). The VAK Survey, developed by Walter Burke Barbe and Neil Fleming, asks a series of questions. Again, remember this is only to raise your *awareness* of your preferences, not dictate how you should learn.

What many people find is that they like to take in information in a multitude of ways but they do notice they are more distracted during particular methods of learning. Noticing these *sensitivities* might be another insight for you.

Learning Style Assessment

Visual, Auditory, and Kinesthetic Survey

Read each statement carefully. To the left of each statement, write the number that best describes how each statement applies to you, using the following guide:

1	2	3	4	5
Almost Never Applies	Applies Once In A While	Sometimes Applies	Often Applies	Almost Always Applies

There are no correct or incorrect answers. Trust your gut and enter what comes to mind first for you.

Once you have completed all 36 statements (12 statements in three sections), total your score in the spaces provided.

Section One – Visual

_____ 1. I take lots of notes and I like to doodle.

_____ 2. When talking to someone else I have a hard time if they don't maintain good eye contact with me.

_____ 3. I make lists and notes because I remember things better if I write them down.

_____ 4. When reading a novel I pay a lot of attention to passages describing the clothing, objects, scenery, setting, etc.

_____ 5. I need to write down directions in order to remember them.

_____ 6. I need to see the person I am talking to keep focused on the subject.

_____ 7. When meeting a person for the first time I notice their style of dress, visual characteristics, and how they're "put together" first.

_____ 8. When I am at a party, one of the things I love to do is stand back and "people-watch."

_____ 9. When recalling information, I can see it in my mind and remember where I saw it.

_____ 10. If I had to explain a new procedure or technique, I would prefer to write it out.

_____ 11. In my free time, I am most likely to watch television or read.

_____ 12. If someone has a message for me, I am most comfortable when they send it in a written format.

Total For Visual _____ (note: the minimum is 12 and maximum is 60)

Section Two – Auditory

_____ 1. When I read, I read out loud or move my lips to hear the words in my head.

_____ 2. When talking to someone else I have a hard time staying engaged with those who do not talk back with me.

_____ 3. I do not take a lot of notes but I still remember what was said. Taking notes distracts me from the speaker.

_____ 4. When reading a novel I pay a lot of attention to passages involving conversations, talking, speaking, dialogues, etc.

_____ 5. I like to talk to myself when solving a problem or writing.

_____ 6. I can understand what a speaker says, even if I am not focused on the speaker.

_____ 7. I remember things easier by repeating them again and again.

_____ 8. When I am at a party, one of the things I love to do is talk in-depth about a subject that is important to me with a good conversationalist.

_____ 9. I would rather receive information from the radio, rather than a newspaper.

_____ 10. If I had to explain a new procedure or technique, I would prefer telling about it.

_____ 11. With free time I am most likely to listen to music.

_____ 12. If someone has a message for me, I am most comfortable if they call on the phone.

Total For Auditory _____ (note: the minimum is 12 and maximum is 60)

Section Three - Kinesthetic

_____ 1. I am not good at reading or listening to directions. I would rather just start working on the task or project at hand.

_____ 2. When talking to someone else I have a hard time if they don't show any kind of emotional support.

_____ 3. I take notes and doodle but I rarely go back and look at them.

_____ 4. When reading a novel I pay a lot of attention to passages revealing feelings, moods, action, drama, etc.

_____ 5. When I am reading, I move my lips.

_____ 6. I will exchange words and places and use my hands a lot when I can't remember the right thing to say.

_____ 7. My desk appears disorganized.

_____ 8. When I am at a party, one of the things I love to do is activities such as dancing, games, and totally losing myself in the action.

_____ 9. I like to move around. I feel trapped when seated at a meeting or a desk.

_____ 10. If I had to explain a new procedure or technique, I would prefer to demonstrate it.

_____ 11. With free time I am most likely to exercise.

_____ 12. If someone has a message for me, I am most comfortable if they talk to me in person.

Total For Kinesthetic _____ (note: the minimum is 12 and maximum is 60)

SCORING PROCEDURE

Total each section and place the sum in the blocks below:

VISUAL	AUDITORY	KINESTHETIC
number of points: _____	number of points: _____	number of points: _____

The area in which you have the highest score represents your best learning style. See big numbers in EVERY box? That means you engage with ALL three styles, but you probably learn best using one style.

Visual Learners

If you are a visual learner, you learn by reading or seeing pictures. You understand and remember things by sight. You can picture what you are learning in your head, and you learn best by primarily visual methods. You like to see what you are learning.

As a visual learner, you are usually neat and clean. You often close your eyes to visualize or remember something, and you will find something to watch if you become bored. You may have difficulty with spoken directions and be easily distracted by sounds. You are attracted to color and spoken language (like stories) rich in imagery.

Here are some things that visual learners like you can do to learn better:
- Sit near the front of the classroom. (It won't mean you're the teacher's pet!)
- Have your eyesight checked on a regular basis.
- Use flashcards to learn new words.
- Try to visualize things that you hear or things that are read to you.
- Write down key words, ideas, or instructions.
- Draw pictures to help explain new concepts and then explain the pictures.
- Color code things.
- Avoid distractions during study times.

Remember that you need to see things, not just hear things, to learn well.

Auditory Learners

If you are an auditory learner, you learn by hearing and listening. You understand and remember things you have heard. You store information by how it sounds and have an easier time understanding spoken instructions than written ones. You often learn by reading out loud because you must hear or speak it to know it.

As an auditory learner, you probably hum or talk to yourself or others if you're bored. People may think you are not paying attention, even though you may be hearing and understanding everything being said.

Here are some things auditory learners like you can do to learn better:
- Sit where you can hear.
- Have your hearing checked on a regular basis.
- Use flashcards to learn new words; read them out loud.
- Read stories, assignments, or directions out loud.
- Record yourself spelling words and then listen to the recording.
- Have test questions read to you out loud.
- Study new material by reading it out loud.

Remember that you need to hear things, not just see things, to learn well.

Kinesthetic Learners

If you are a kinesthetic (aka tactile) learner, you learn by touching and doing. You understand and remember things through physical movement. You are a "hands-on" learner who prefers to touch, move, build, or draw what you learn, and you tend to learn better when some type of physical activity is involved. You need to be active and take frequent breaks. You often speak with your hands and with gestures, and you may have difficulty sitting still.

As a tactile learner, you like to take things apart and put them together, and you tend to find reasons to tinker or move around when you're bored. You may be very well coordinated and have good athletic ability. You can easily remember things that were done but may have difficulty remembering what you saw or heard. You often communicate by touching and appreciate physically expressed forms of encouragement, such as a pat on the back.

Here are some things that tactile learners like you can do to learn better:
- Participate in activities that involve touching, building, moving, or drawing.
- Do lots of hands-on activities like completing art projects, taking walks, or acting out stories.
- It's okay to chew gum, walk around, or rock in a chair while reading or studying.
- Use flashcards and arrange them in groups to show relationships between ideas.
- Trace words with your finger to learn spelling (finger spelling).
- Take frequent breaks during reading or studying periods (frequent, but not long).
- It's okay to tap a pencil, shake your foot, or hold on to something while learning.
- Use a computer to reinforce learning through the sense of touch.

Remember that you learn best by doing, not just by reading, seeing, or hearing.

Access this and all other forms online at https://doula-training.carriekenner.com/doula-assessment-forms-book

Your Learning Style(s)

Learner Sensitivities

Knowing your preferred learning style can help you focus on how to take in new information. But knowing what derails your learning can be equally important. Answer the questions below to see what makes you susceptible to distraction, interrupting your learning flow, and the connections your brain and body are trying to make.

Using the same scale from above, write the number that best describes how each statement applies to you by using the following guide:

1	2	3	4	5
Almost Never Applies	Applies Once In A While	Sometimes Applies	Often Applies	Almost Always Applies

What do you find most distracting when you're learning (either in a course or studying on your own):

_____ People walking by
_____ Noises from outside (mowers, people talking, traffic)
_____ Music in the background
_____ Poor video quality
_____ Lights too bright or too dim
_____ An uncomfortable chair
_____ The temperature being too hot or too cold
_____ Poorly organized or edited handouts
_____ Other students' comments and questions

There's no need to total your scores for this section. Just notice the variables above that have a 3, 4, or 5 rating.

It can be tempting to try to connect your sensitivities to your learning style but you don't need to over-complicate things. Simply use the data above to **create a learning environment that best suits your learning preferences** and avoids as many distractions as possible.

For example, if an uncomfortable chair is a big problem for you and you're attending an in-person training where you have no control over the quality of chairs, contact the instructor to ask if you can bring your own. Some people in my in-person trainings chose to sit on upright cushioned chairs, using backjacks on the floor, in their own camp chair, or draped over a physioball. (And, while you're at it, bring many layers of clothing to adapt to changing room temperatures.)

If visual distractions are a problem for you, sit with your back to the window, hallway, or door.

If sounds bug you, sit near the front in an in-person training, or attend an online training in a closed room or wearing noise-canceling headphones.

If there are many variables that bother you—sounds, lights, chairs, and temperature—even if you'd prefer an in-person training, consider an online course where you can control more of those variables.

If you are sensitive to the quality of presentations or materials, ask for a sample handout or video to see if a course will work for you.

CHAPTER 12

Know Your Training Options

When it comes to doula trainings, there are many options to choose from:

» Online or in person

» A few days in a row, a weekly series, or spread out over months

» Scheduled sessions or self-paced modules

» Or no training at all!

The problem is, you don't have a lot of money or time to invest in a training that won't do a good job of preparing you to be a doula, or to get partway through your training only to find out it's not a good fit for your learning style. That's why I'm going to help you learn all about doula trainings— so you won't have to make any costly mistakes.

As a highly experienced doula trainer, I believe there's a way to set up a training that delivers the best results for students. I'm going to show you how I structure my courses and the way I deliver content, so you understand what to look for in a training.

The Anatomy of a Great Doula Training

A doula training should include explanations, demonstrations, and exercises to develop the basic skills of being a doula, like the ones I outlined in Chapter 10. You should be able to understand the *why* and the *how* for each skill. In addition, a comprehensive training should include the following components:

A historical timeline that moves from the past to the present to the future—The history of the doula role, the history of your field, and what problems clients currently face and how they can be improved by the presence of a doula.

An exploration of the social context that you'll be working in—The larger social context of where you and your clients live, the individual system(s) within your chosen field, and the specific scenarios in which you'll be working.

Industry-specific knowledge—The technical or detailed knowledge of the systems, facilities, processes, procedures, and personnel involved in your industry or field. This may include specific skills that will be needed to support the clients you will be working with.

The emotional terrain—An exploration of the emotional experience that people have when moving through this life event, and the transformative aspects that may be experienced. The potential for psychological and/or spiritual experiences should be discussed.

Relaxation, stress-reduction, and/or comfort techniques—Depending on your field, you should learn tools to help clients (and you) manage stress, develop relaxation strategies, and use hands-on comfort techniques like appropriate touch, hand massage, and movements. It's an added bonus if your training includes modalities such as aromatherapy, visualization, guided meditations, and somatic practices.

Decision-making tools—The communication techniques and assessment tools that you can use to help your clients with the decision-making process before, during, and after their life event. Client advocacy and empowerment strategies should also be discussed.

Situational examples—An outline of common situations and experiences that your clients may have, typical challenges or problems that clients will face, and how to manage complex cases that may arise in your industry or field.

I believe a good doula training will also include crucial information on the intersections of racism, marginalization, and oppression within your field; teach the material and strategies through a trauma-informed lens; and provide opportunities for self-reflection and personal growth throughout the educational process.

Finally, the material should be presented in a variety of ways to meet the needs of various learners. I had a motto as an in-person teacher: "Say it three ways. Show it three ways (printed word, demo, illustration). And receive it three ways (video, audio, written)." Make sure your doula training offers content via video, audio, print, illustrations, graphs, demonstrations, and interactive methods.

I offer *Become a Doula: Foundational Training for All Types of Doulas*, which is a perfect start for any kind of doula. It provides a historical, social, and political review of the doula movement, comprehensive training in all of the primary doula skills, with an emphasis on my area of expertise: communication, relaxation and comfort techniques, and decision-making support skills.

If you already have experience in your field, this may be all the training you need to get started. And if you know you want a specialty training for your doula role, but aren't quite ready to dive in, *Become a Doula: Foundational Training for All Types of Doulas* is a great way to dip your toes in the water first..

The world is your oyster, doulas. Let's get started with finding out the format of training that will work best for you...

Doula Training Formats

Where you go to get trained: In-person or virtual (online)

How long you have to complete it: Time-bound (has predetermined start and end dates) or self-paced

Time frame it's delivered in: Intensive (a few days) or spread out over time (for example, twelve weeks or nine months, etc.)

How information is delivered: Live, pre-recorded, or a combination; video modules; digital handouts; printed material

Interaction with instructor(s): In live sessions, scheduled calls, or not at all

Interaction with other students: Cohort-based or discussion groups

Features of a Training Program

Now that you understand the key differences between training programs, it's time to learn about the features within a program that may matter to you as well. Each training program will feature:

The amount of content: How many hours of live teaching, videos, reading, and/or homework is offered or required?

How the material is accessed: Can you download it? Access it online only? Are books required?

How content is available: Are all modules available at once, dripped out over time, or are you required to complete one module before moving on to the next? How long can you access it? If you miss an in-person session, how can you make it up?

How comprehensive is the course: Does it cover basic doula skills, advanced doula skills, technical information for the doula role, technical information for the field you're in, business skills, interpersonal skills, or other areas you are interested in?

Does it offer or require tests or quizzes: Yes/no, how many, are they required to move on to the next module?

One instructor or many: Do you have access to one person only or a team of instructors or coaches?

Philosophy: Does the program or instructor have a value-based underpinning that infuses the training, such as BIPOC-led, reproductive justice focus, Christian based, steeped in African traditions or Indigenous practices, gender inclusive, based on the Sacred Feminine, holistic, uses a healing tradition framework (traditional Chinese medicine, herbalism, ayurvedic, etc.)?

Accessibility: Does the course content support multiple learning styles (written, spoken, visuals, demonstrations, etc.)? Does it include captions and transcripts?

Cost of Training

Doula trainings can range from hundreds to thousands of dollars. You may find the training you want to take most but can't afford it. I'll show you how to balance out what you *want* to do with what you *can* do in the next chapter. But for now, here's what you need to know about the cost of doula trainings:

Longer programs tend to cost more than shorter or immersive programs: It can be helpful to estimate the overall hours of content you are getting for the price—and the quality of that content—to determine if the higher price is worth it to you.

Payment plans may be available to spread payments over many months: Many training programs offer payment plans. This option may have additional fees attached, but smaller payments over time make it attainable for more people. Note that in some programs, course content may be limited until you have paid in full, while in other programs it is not.

Many doula trainings offer scholarships for marginalized or historically oppressed people: Some scholarships are need based, and some are equity based. Look at scholarship requirements (forms, writing, deadlines, amounts, etc.) before deciding if a scholarship is a potential solution for you.

The cost doesn't necessarily reflect the quality of the program: You're going to learn how to assess the quality of a program (to some extent) in the next chapter. For now, I want you to know that there are three factors for determining quality: 1) the experience of the instructor, both as a working doula and as an instructor; 2) the way the material is delivered (quantity and quality), and 3) the outcomes the course delivers. If your sense is that any of those aren't top-notch, a program isn't worth top dollar.

There's the price *of the training, and the entire* cost *to take it:* In addition to the price you see posted on a website, you need to factor in the cost of required books or materials, childcare, or missed work. If you are traveling to attend a training, also factor in transportation costs; accommodations and meals; missed income; expenses to care for children, pets, or others in your absence; and any other expenses that you'll incur to attend the training.

Low-risk investments: A mini-course to get you started or a book (like my upcoming book *Becoming a Birth Doula,* which will be published in 2025). There are also alternatives to formal training programs, such as apprenticeships, internships, and self-study.

If the cost of taking a formal training is unrealistic for you, consider an alternative. Just remember that they may not be entirely free, and you will need to make sure you meet any regulatory, certification, or licensing requirements in your area if you take an alternative path.

Certification

Certification is a hot topic in many doula fields. In the birth doula world, certification was considered the gold standard for many years. More recently, birth doula certification is viewed as entirely optional and in some cases looked down upon. Today's doulas need to decide if certification is important to them—or required for the way they want to work—and make sure the training program they take will meet their certification needs.

So what does doula certification look like?

Certification usually consists of the doula completing a formal training program (often the training offered by the certifying body), serving a certain number of clients, receiving positive evaluations from clients and/or other professionals in the field, getting a character reference, doing a self-evaluation, and perhaps taking continuing education. Some certification programs simply require the doula to complete the training program and they are automatically certified.

The doula submits their certification documents and then an individual or panel of experienced doulas approves or denies their certification. They get a certificate and maybe a name badge and digital badge for their website and—*voila!*—they are now certified.

Certification may need to be renewed every year or two or three (kinda silly, since most doulas don't *lose* skills over time). Many organizations offer lifetime certification.

There are two primary benefits to certification:

1. For the doula, they know they've met a standard of professionalism that is meaningful to them. The certification process will typically help them hone their skills and feel confident they are providing quality care. These doulas proudly announce their certification to the world.

2. For the client, they know their doula has met a standard of care by a certifying body. Realistically, they rarely know what that standard is, or anything about the certifying body. So besides the badge on the doula's website, certification is pretty meaningless to consumers. In my fifteen years practicing as a birth doula, not one client asked if I was certified.

Oh wait, there's one more benefit... for certifying organizations. Certification processing and renewals are a source of income.

The bottom-line question for most doulas is: *Do I have to be certified to practice as a doula?* The answer varies greatly from field to field, state to state, and often location to location. Here are the questions and answers you'll need to find for your field:

Is certification *legally* required? At the state level, some professionals are required *by law* to be licensed or registered by the state in order to practice legally. Licensing and registration may stipulate approved training programs, require you to pass a test, submit special forms, attend additional training, get certification by an organization or board, and pay a fee. An example of licensed professions are massage therapists, midwives, and psychotherapists. Registered professionals (in my state) include nurses and counselors. At the time of this publication, no states require any type of doulas to be licensed or registered to practice legally.

Can a facility require me to be certified? Some hospitals may require birth doulas to be certified, though hospitals aren't equipped to screen or enforce this. During the COVID pandemic, many hospitals implemented this requirement. Instead of keeping non-certified doulas out (and for what purpose?), those doulas just created doula certification programs and certified themselves. There is no official clearinghouse for "approved" doula certifications. Yes, facilities can implement their own rules for who can enter or not, but these are not legal issues and can often be worked around.

Who else might require certification? Third-party-funded doula programs often require certification because they aren't equipped to assess doula qualification on their own. State-run programs that pay for doulas to support families on Medicaid, or nonprofits that receive grants to pay doulas to serve low-income clients, don't know anything about doula training, so they require the doulas in their program to be certified. Hospital-based doula programs or doula agencies may require certification as one of the screening tools before hiring doulas to their teams. I know quite a few doulas who got certified just so they could join a program or agency.

Recently, some states have seen lawsuits that require death doulas to be licensed as funeral directors to practice legally (the suits failed). I'm sure other doula roles will be targeted for certification, licensing, or regulatory requirements as well. When doulas are seen as a threat to established entities, they may be challenged by people who don't understand their role. But when doulas adhere to non-clinical, non-technical roles, they are safe from legal harassment. At least for now.

So if anyone can create certification and it's no big deal to obtain it, why don't all doulas just get certified? The downside of certification is that the certifying organization may have guidelines, a scope of practice, rules, or dues that the doula doesn't agree with. Certification is also patriarchal, hierarchical, and part of the rule-based tenets of white supremacy that many people want no part of.

I know doulas who have practiced for dozens of years who aren't certified but they are extremely qualified. So doula certification should be an option for those who are interested or need it, but not required. Please consider this so you can find a training that will support your intentions.

Now it's time to see which doula training formats and features appeal to you. To find out what kind of training you are most interested in, complete the Doula Training Preferences sheet.

DOULA TRAINING PREFERENCES

This tool is designed to list all the features you may find in a doula training, and identify your preferences for each.

Check the box for all statements you agree with below:

LOCATION
- ☐ I prefer an in-person training
- ☐ I prefer an online training

LENGTH OF TRAINING
- ☐ I prefer an intensive course (a few days in a row)
- ☐ I prefer regular classes spanning weeks or months
- ☐ I want my training to be on-going or unlimited

TIME TO COMPLETE
- ☐ I want a training that is time bound (specific start/end dates)
- ☐ I want a training that is self-paced so I can go as fast or slow as I want

INFORMATION PROVIDED
- ☐ I want all the information provided live (in person or virtual)
- ☐ I'd like pre-recorded training videos
- ☐ I like lots of digital handouts I can download
- ☐ I like printed materials given or sent to me

INTERACTION WITH INSTRUCTORS
- ☐ I want to meet with my instructor in live sessions (in person or virtual)
- ☐ I'd like at least monthly calls with my instructor
- ☐ I'd like to interact with my instructor in an online chat group
- ☐ I don't need any interaction with the instructor

NUMBER OF INSTRUCTORS
- ☐ I'm fine with just one instructor
- ☐ I want a team of instructors I can learn from
- ☐ I want a team of instructors I can interact with
- ☐ I'd like one main instructor and a team of coaches to ask questions with

INTERACTION WITH OTHER STUDENTS

- ☐ I want to meet other students in live sessions (in person or virtual)
- ☐ I'd like at least monthly calls to interact with other students
- ☐ I'd like to interact with other students in an online chat group
- ☐ I'd like a specific cohort of students I get to know
- ☐ I'd like to interact with any other students who've taken this course
- ☐ I don't need any interaction with other students

HOW TO ACCESS MATERIAL

- ☐ I want materials I can download
- ☐ It's okay if I can only access material online
- ☐ I'm fine having to buy additional books
- ☐ I want material dripped out over time so I don't get overwhelmed
- ☐ I want access to material all at once so I can go through it when I want
- ☐ I want to be required to finish one module before going on to the next
- ☐ I want lifetime access to the material

COMPREHENSIVENESS OF THE COURSE

- ☐ I want my training to cover basic doula skills and information for my field
- ☐ I want my training to include technical information for my field
- ☐ I want my training to include advanced doula skills for my field
- ☐ I want my doula training to include interpersonal skills for doulas
- ☐ I want my training to include business skills for starting my career
- ☐ I want my training to include complementary skills like energy work, bodywork, NLP, stress management

TEST OR QUIZZES

- ☐ I want my training to include quizzes to test what I'm learning as I go
- ☐ I want my training to test me before I can go on to the next module
- ☐ I want one test at the end of the training
- ☐ I don't want any testing!

ACCESSIBILITY	
☐	I want or need closed captions on videos
☐	I want or need transcripts of videos
☐	I like audio-only presentations
☐	I'd like techniques and skills to be demonstrated, not just described
COST OF TRAINING	
☐	I will pay less than $200 for a training
☐	I will pay up to $500 for a training
☐	I will pay up to $800 for a training
☐	I will pay up to $1000 for a training
☐	I will pay up to $1500 for a training
☐	I will pay over $1500 for a training

Access this and all other forms online at https://doula-training.carriekenner.com/doula-assessment-forms-book

CHAPTER 13

Researching Doula Trainings

Now that you have a sense of what kind of training you think you'd enjoy most, it's time to dive in and start looking at some specific options for your chosen doula field. You may have many to choose from, or only a few. Or, you may have to create your own process for becoming a doula if there's no formal training available or suitable for you.

Some of the key things to look for are:

- Is the training in person or online?
- Is it time-bound or self-paced?
- What topics does it include?
- What is the cost?

How to Research Doula Trainings Online

You're going to need access to the internet to look for doula trainings. You could schedule a few hours to do this preliminary research, or take fifteen minutes each morning, lunch period, or evening to look at one or two at a time until you feel "done."

Follow the steps below to start gathering information. Keep notes of which trainings you find, write down what appeals to you (or doesn't) for each, and start the process of narrowing your choices to the top three, which you will research in detail in the next chapter.

> Here are a few things to look (and watch out) for when researching doula trainings:
> - » Read the About page: Do you like what you see?
> - » Who is the instructor or founders? What's their story?
> - » Why did they start a doula training? When did they start it?
> - » What kind of lived experience as a doula do they have? Do they talk about both the rewards and challenges of being a doula?
> - » What kind of teaching experience do they have? Do they train for an organization or for themselves? Did they teach anything before launching a doula training?
> - » Are they focused on one area, a few fields, or all they all over the place? Do they seem focused or scattered?
> - » Are they active in their community or region as an ambassador for doulas? Do they speak to the politics of being a doula?
> - » Do they offer sample classes, info sessions, or videos to see what their presence is like?

> » What makes their doula training stand out or seem unique compared to other trainings?
>
> » How can you contact them if you have questions or problems?
>
> » What is their refund policy?
>
> These questions will help you peek behind the curtain for a sense of their longevity, authority, professionalism, and style.'

Step 1:

Do an internet search using phrases like "[your field] doula training near me." If you are open to online training, you can omit the "near me" part.

Step 2:

Read all the pages on the website. As you read, enter the information on the Training Tracking Sheet. Try to be open-minded and objective as you learn about each training program. Just capture the information on the tracking sheet, knowing you will assess them later.

Step 3:

Contact the training organization if you have further questions.

Step 4:

When you feel you have looked at enough trainings to satisfy your curiosity, continue to the next chapter.

Use this tracking sheet to keep notes on the training format and features:

SO YOU WANT TO BE A DOULA

TRAINING TRACKING SHEET

1. Do an internet search using phrases like "[your field, such as birth, death, divorce, etc.)] doula training near me." If you are open to online training, you can omit the "near me" part or "online" to your search.

2. Read all the pages on the website. As you read, enter their information in this Training Tracking Sheet. Try to be open-minded and objective as you learn about each training program. Just capture the information below, knowing you will assess them later.

3. Contact the training organization if you have further questions.

	TRAINING PROGRAM 1	TRAINING PROGRAM 2	TRAINING PROGRAM 3	TRAINING PROGRAM 4	TRAINING PROGRAM 5
NAME OF TRAINING PROGRAM >>					
LOCATION					
In Person					
Virtual					
LENGTH OF COURSE					
Intensive (few days)					
Weeks-Months					
Unlimited					
CONTENT					
All live					
All pre-recorded					
Combination					
TIME TO COMPLETE					
Specific start-end dates					
Self-paced					
INSTRUCTOR INTERACTION					
Live training sessions					
Live Q&A sessions					
Online chat group					
None					

Researching Doula Trainings

	TRAINING PROGRAM 1	TRAINING PROGRAM 2	TRAINING PROGRAM 3	TRAINING PROGRAM 4	TRAINING PROGRAM 5
STUDENT INTERACTIONS					
Live with my cohort					
Additional calls					
Online chat group					
None					
TIME COMMITMENT					
# hours of live sessions					
# hours of videos					
# hours of homework					
MATERIALS					
Downloadable					
Access online only					
Required books to buy					
DRIP SCHEDULE FOR ONLINE COURSES					
Content dripped out over time					
Content available all at once					
Must complete one module before going on to next one					
COMPREHENSIVENESS					
Basic doula skills					
Technical information for my field					
Advanced doula skills					
Business skills					
Interpersonal skills					
Complementary skills					

SO YOU WANT TO BE A DOULA

	TRAINING PROGRAM 1	TRAINING PROGRAM 2	TRAINING PROGRAM 3	TRAINING PROGRAM 4	TRAINING PROGRAM 5
TEST/QUIZZES					
# of tests					
Tests optional					
Test required					
Test at end					
No tests					
INSTRUCTORS					
# of instructors					
# of coaches					
PHILOSOPHY					
BIPOC-led					
Reproductive Justice					
African Traditions					
Indigenous Practices					
Inclusive					
Muslim					
Jewish					
Christian					
Sacred Feminine					
Holistic					
Healing framework					
ACCESSIBILITY					
Closed captioned videos					
Transcripts					
Audio files					
Skill demos					

Researching Doula Trainings

	TRAINING PROGRAM 1	TRAINING PROGRAM 2	TRAINING PROGRAM 3	TRAINING PROGRAM 4	TRAINING PROGRAM 5
COST					
Cost of training					
Payment plan options					
Scholarships					
Travel costs					
CERTIFICATION					
Offers certification					
Approved for certification elsewhere					
INTUITION					
On a scale of 0-5, how strong is your intuition to take this training					
EXCITABILITY FACTOR					
On a scale of 0-5, how excited do you get when thinking about this training?					

Access this and all other forms online at https://doula-training.carriekenner.com/doula-assessment-forms-book

CHAPTER 14

Your Top Three Training Options

Now you are going to identify your top three trainings and establish your priorities to determine the one you want to attend. It may not be a clear-cut decision, so now is a good time to put your doula intuition into practice.

Step 1:

Look at your Training Tracking Sheet. Cross off the trainings that do not appeal to you.

Step 2:

Using your gut instincts, notice the trainings that appeal to you the most. Highlight them.

Step 3:

If you highlighted more than three trainings, either select the three most diverse trainings or the three most similar trainings (whichever you are most interested in comparing) and cross the rest off your list.

Step 4:

Establish your training priorities.

Your Training Priorities

Consider these key training formats and features, and decide which are most important to you:

- Location (online or in person)
- Length of course (days, weeks, months, or unlimited)
- Content (live or pre-recorded)
- Time to complete (time-bound or self-paced)
- Instructor interaction
- Student interaction
- Comprehensiveness
- Philosophy
- Cost
- Certification

Now, order them from most important (1) to least important (10) in the spaces below.

1. _____
2. _____
3. _____
4. _____
5. _____
6. _____
7. _____
8. _____

Your Top Three Training Options

9. _____

10. _____

Enter your priority number in the first column to the left of the format or feature in the Find-a-Training Tool.

SO YOU WANT TO BE A DOULA

FIND-A-TRAINING TOOL

#1 Name of Training Program: Website address:
#2 Name of Training Program: Website address:
#3 Name of Training Program: Website address:

INSTRUCTIONS:

1. Enter your priority numbers (1-10) in the first column next to the format or features you prioritized.
2. Using the information from your Training Tracking Sheet, put an 'X' to the right of each variable the training includes.
Add additional information in the 'Notes' column. Do this for each of the three trainings.
3. Starting with priority #1, circle the **one** training in that row which most closely meets your preference. Choose only 1 even if you have to draw straws.
4. Continue with priorities 2-10, circling the **one** training in that row which most closely meets your preference for that format or feature.
5. Add up how many circles each training received and enter that number in the bottom row.
6. Rank the trainings from 1 to 3 for how strong is your intuition to take this training
7. Rank the trainings from 1 to 3 for how excited you get when thinking about this training

Enter your priority numbers here: *Enter an "X" for each variable that applies to the training program in these columns:*

	FORMAT / FEATURE	#1	#1 NOTES	#2	#2 NOTES	#3	#3 NOTES
	LOCATION						
	In Person						
	Virtual						
	LENGTH OF COURSE						
	Intensive (few days)						
	Weeks-Months						
	Unlimited						
	CONTENT						
	All live						
	All pre-recorded						
	Combination						
	TIME TO COMPLETE						
	Specific start-end dates						
	Self-paced						
	INSTRUCTOR INTERACTION						
	Live training sessions						
	Live Q&A sessions						
	Online chat group						
	None						
	STUDENT INTERACTION						
	Live with my cohort						
	Additional calls						
	Online chat group						
	None						
	TIME COMMITMENT						
	# of hours of live sessions						
	# of hours of videos						
	# of hours of homework						
	MATERIAL						
	Downloadable						
	Access online only						
	Required books to buy						

Your Top Three Training Options

Enter your priority numbers here: ↓ *Enter an "X" for each variable that applies to the training program in these columns:* ↓ ↓ ↓

FORMAT / FEATURE	#1	#1 NOTES	#2	#2 NOTES	#3	#3 NOTES
RELEASE SCHEDULE FOR ONLINE COURSES						
Content dripped out over time						
Content avail at once						
Must complete one module before proceed						
COMPREHENSIVENESS						
Basic doula skills						
Technical info for my field						
Advanced doula skills						
Business skills						
Interpersonal skills						
Complementary skills						
TESTS/QUIZZES						
# of tests						
Tests optional						
Test required						
Test at end						
No tests						
INSTRUCTORS						
# of instructors						
# of coaches						
PHILOSOPHY						
BIPOC-led						
Reproductive Justice						
African Traditions						
Indigenous Practices						
Inclusive						
Muslim						
Jewish						
Christian						
Sacred Feminine						
Holistic						
Healing framework						
ACCESSIBILITY						
Closed captioned videos						
Transcripts						
Audio files						
Skill demos						
COST						
Cost of training						
Payment plan options						
Scholarships						
Travel costs						
CERTIFICATION						
Offers certification						
Approved for cert. elsewhere						
		< TOTAL # OF CIRCLES		< TOTAL # OF CIRCLES		< TOTAL # OF CIRCLES

		#1	#1 NOTES	#2	#2 NOTES	#3	#3 NOTES
INTUITION		↓ Enter 1, 2, or 3 here		↓ Enter 1, 2, or 3 here		↓ Enter 1, 2, or 3 here	
Rank the trainings from 1 (weakest) to 3 (strongest) for how strong is your intuition to take this training							
EXCITABILITY FACTOR		↓ Enter 1, 2, or 3 here		↓ Enter 1, 2, or 3 here		↓ Enter 1, 2, or 3 here	
Rank the trainings from 1 (least) to 3 (most) for how excited you get when thinking about this training							

Add the *total number of circles with the two numbers above* in the boxes below:

[ ] < TOTAL SCORE   [ ] < TOTAL SCORE   [ ] < TOTAL SCORE

Congratulations! You've found the winner! *The training with the highest score "wins."*

What if you don't like the result? That's okay. This is an exercise designed to activate both your objective thinking mind *and* your intuition. If the objective process doesn't sit well with you, by all means listen to your intuition. If you don't trust your intuition, use the objective results.

Access this and all other forms online at https://doula-training.carriekenner.com/doula-assessment-forms-book

Using the information from your Training Tracking Sheet, fill in the information for your top three choices. I know you did it already, but **doing it again will help you think about it more deeply.** This time, you have more information to compare. You have more clarity on your priorities. You know so much more about doula trainings than when you started.

A few things to keep in mind as you consider your top three choices:

- Be realistic about the time commitment each training will require.

- Be sure to consider ALL costs—the training itself, plus extra books or materials; time off from work; cost of child, pet, or home care while you attend the training; cost of travel, lodging, and meals away from home.

- When you weigh your priorities, it will be easier to choose between how the training is delivered or the charisma of the trainer or the focus of the content. There is plenty of time in the future to get additional information or study with stellar trainers.

Step 1:

Enter your priority numbers (1-10) in the first column next to the format or features you prioritized.

Step 2:

Using the information from your Training Tracking Sheet, put an 'X' to the right of each variable the training includes. Add additional information in the 'Notes' column. Do this for each of the three trainings.

Step 3:

Starting with priority #1, circle the one training in that row which most closely meets your preference. Choose only 1 even if you have to draw straws.

Step 4:

Continue with priorities 2-10, circling the one training in that row which most closely meets your preference for that format or feature.

Step 5:

Add up how many circles each training received and enter that number in the bottom row.

Step 6:

Rank the trainings from 1 to 3 for how strong is your intuition to take this training

Step 7:

Rank the trainings from 1 to 3 for how excited you get when thinking about this training

Step 8:

Add up the Total Number of Circles, the Intuition ranking, and the Excitability Factor ranking for each column.

The training that received the most circles "wins."

But what if you don't like the result? That's okay. This is an exercise designed to activate both your objective-thinking mind *and* your intuition. If the objective process doesn't sit well with you, by all means listen to your intuition. If you don't trust your intuition, use the objective results.

Remember: Your doula training is not the end-all be-all o your education. You'll really learn how to be a doula when you are working with clients, so don't let finding the "perfect" training hold you up.

SO YOU WANT TO BE A DOULA

By now, you should have your top choice for a doula training. Congratulations!

Next step: Register for your training and get started!

CHAPTER 15

How to Fund Your Doula Training

Many aspiring doulas don't have extra money sitting around for a doula training. If that's you, here are some helpful ideas for how to fund your training:

Step 1:

Create a budget so you know how much you actually need. Include the following items:

Cost of the training	$
Cost of additional materials (books and supplies)	$
Cost of missed work (# of hours x hourly wage)	$
Cost of child, pet, elder, or house-sitting while you are attending the training or doing homework (# of hours x caregiver rate)	$
Travel costs (gas, transit fares, Uber, airfare, parking, etc.)	$
Lodging costs for out-of-town training	$

Meals while at training	$_____
Total cost of training:	$_____

Step 2:

Next, where can you cut some of those costs? Are any books or materials available to borrow from a library, friend, or someone in your doula community? Can you trade childcare with a neighbor? Can you bring your lunch? Identify any areas where you can save money, and make a list to see if those things are available. If so, cross them off your budget. See, you're saving money already!

Step 3:

Get creative.

- Make a list of people who have said "You'd make such a great doula!" or were excited when you told them about becoming a doula, and ask them to donate to your doula training fund. This may feel uncomfortable, but I promise you, people want to help other people do good things if they can. The worst that can happen is they say they can't help you out right now.
- If you have a birthday or holiday coming up, ask for money for the doula training in lieu of gifts.
- Ask a friend to loan you the money and create a payback plan.
- If you have a credit card, charge it.
- Start a GoFundMe campaign to raise funds.

Step 4:

Ask the training organization if they have scholarships, payment plans, or work-trade opportunities. Most do.

Step 5:

If there are doula community organizations in your area, or organizations that serve your clientele, ask if they have scholarships or grants available that you can apply for. They may require you to work for them in exchange, but it may be a great way to get your training paid for and get your first clients.

Step 6:

Start saving. Create a savings plan and start putting away as much each week as you can afford. Try these fun saving ideas:

- See if your bank has a "round up" function on debit card purchases. For every purchase you make, it automatically rounds up the figure to the nearest dollar amount and puts the "change" into a savings account. If your bank doesn't do this, consider paying cash for things (I know, so old school!) and always use paper money to pay. Put all your change into a container at the end of the day and watch it fill up.

- Choose one thing you buy daily (coffee or snacks) and start bringing them from home. Take what you normally would have spent on them each day and put it into a savings jar. Watch it fill up.

- Open an extra savings account and have an amount automatically deducted from your paycheck deposited each pay period. Watch it fill up.

- Cancel one of your streaming or membership services and put that money in a savings account instead.

Step 7:

Do some extra things to earn money just for your doula training. Take on a part-time job, mow lawns on the weekend, do household tasks for a neighbor, work a few extra hours a week— you get the idea. Figure out how many hours you'll need at the rate of pay, and set a time frame so you don't get burned out.

The passion you have for becoming a doula will likely be met in equal measure by sources that want to support you. Turn your passion into energy—and that energy into money—and you'll soon be on your way.

CHAPTER 16

Alternatives to Formal Doula Training

If no training is available for your chosen doula role, or the training options aren't suitable for you, you can still become a doula. You just might have to get a little more creative and find a mentor, or create your own training process. Here's how:

Think back to the family and community support that people traditionally relied on during challenging times. Where did the local midwife learn their skills? How did the farmer learn how to integrate a new animal into a flock? How did a preacher know how to counsel someone through grief? Likely by watching others or through apprenticeship.

This approach to training is going to work best for aspiring doulas who are already familiar with their field of interest; either they worked in the industry professionally, or they went through the life event personally. Having this knowledge already means you won't be starting as a total beginner, and it will be easier to access specific information for your role. But it isn't mandatory, so if this is your path, just be sure to include industry-specific learning along with developing your doula skills.

Step 1:

Look for other doulas in your chosen field, and reach out to them to ask if they will mentor you. They could be local or live far away. If you find somebody local, you may be able to "shadow" them and learn by watching and doing. If you don't have somebody near you, they can share their experiences and resources with you. Don't feel bad if you can't find a willing mentor. Some people are generous with their time and expertise, others aren't. Keep looking if you need to, or move on to Step 2.

Step 2:

If there are no other doulas in your field, or if you can't find someone in Step 1 who is willing to help you get started, find a person in your community (or even across the globe if you need to) who has the skills you want to possess. Perhaps they are a professional in your area of interest, or a doula in another field. Maybe you saw them speak or teach a class and wanted to learn their style. The point is to find someone you look up to and want to learn from. Ask them if they would be willing to share their skills with you.

Step 3:

Develop a training plan. What are the skills you need to learn, and how will you learn them? Your "training" could consist of books, one-on-one sessions with your mentor, watching videos, taking online courses, etc. Look for advanced trainings specifically for doulas that could be helpful for you (such as neuro linguistic-programming, acupressure, self-care, managing challenging clients, etc.). Work with your mentor to design your training with specific goals and deadlines. They can coach you through the process and keep you on track, as well as help you find additional resources when you want to learn something else.

Step 4:

If you aren't already knowledgeable about your specific area of interest, offer to volunteer where you'll be working as a doula. Learn the systems, processes, and procedures from the inside. Start talking to other people who work in that field. Find individuals who have gone through this life event and interview them about their experiences. What worked for them? What didn't? What would they have wanted a doula to do for them?

Step 5:

Grow your network. Reach out to other doulas in your community (regardless of their area of expertise). Connect with other professionals in your industry. Constantly be on the lookout for free trainings or community gatherings you can join to learn more and meet others in your field.

You may be wondering if you will have to pay for someone to mentor you. The answer is probably *yes*. You are asking people to devote their time and energy to you, and it is reasonable to reimburse them for that. Consider it a (possibly) lower-cost alternative to a traditional doula training. You may also have to invest some money in a few additional courses or books, but there's also a lot of free resources on YouTube or at the library. So get creative.

Remember, you can combine my *Become a Doula: Foundational Training for All Types of Doulas* course with someone who has expertise in your field to create a solid training program for your doula career.

Tips for Success and Completion

No matter which training path you choose, it can be a lot of work to complete the process. So I'd like to share a few tips for setting yourself up for success.

1. **Budget your money** for the cost of the training and any additional materials you'll need along the way. Set up a special bank account if you need to save the money, or if you want to earmark some funds just for this purpose.

2. **Clear your calendar** of extra activities as much as you can for the duration of your training program. You might shorten your trips to the gym or go fewer times each week. You might get family members to take over all your household chores while you're in study mode. Cut out one social evening a week, or only go to family dinners once a month instead of every weekend. It's only temporary.

3. **Budget your time** so you can fit your training into your current life. Be very realistic and honest with yourself here. If you're taking an in-person course and you have to sit in a classroom for twenty-four hours, you don't have to fit it into your daily life. But if you're taking an online course that includes twenty-five hours of video, five books, and thirty handouts to read, you're looking at nearly one hundred hours of home study.

   Where are those hours going to come from? You likely don't have to read *all* the things at first, but at a minimum, plan to watch all the videos, read a few of the books, and do most of the handouts.

   If you work full time, you'll have to reserve time outside of work for studying. If you have kids, that time is likely not available to you. So maybe you'll be getting up an hour early, or staying up an hour late each day. Or you'll study during your lunch break. Or take six hours every Saturday. However you work it out, **put it on your calendar** and stick to it as best you can.

   Not sticking to a time budget is the most common obstacle to completing a doula training. I've seen it over and over again. So be realistic. If you have six hours a week to complete sixty hours of study, it will take you ten weeks (two and a half months). There is nothing wrong with that. Just plan a fun celebration when you complete the last module—and stay on course.

4. **Keep a list** of additional books, courses, people, websites, articles, etc. you want to learn from in the future. Avoid the "shiny object syndrome" and try to hold off on diving into these resources just yet. Give yourself the gift of just focusing on your training program for now. All the extras will be waiting for you when you're done.

5. **Find a study buddy or accountability partner.** They might be someone in your training program, or a friend. Set up expectations for yourself and each other. You do not have to be following the same timetable at all. Schedule regular check-in sessions and honor them like an important meeting. Encourage each other, problem-solve together, and celebrate

small milestones along the way. Having a buddy can make the process much more fun and way less isolating.

I remember the excitement of starting my doula training, the lifelong friends and connections I made, and the tremendous reward of starting my doula career. I hope you find the same joy and satisfaction in your journey. If you get stuck along the way, visit my website (www.carriekenner.com) to join my online community where you can get encouragement, ideas, support, and camaraderie from other doulas in training. Best wishes to you!

❈ ❈ ❈

Now that you know the doula role and doula training you want to pursue, it's time to think about your future *business* as a doula. Unfortunately, many doula training programs don't include the crucial information on what you need to do after you're trained. I don't want you to take one more step without knowing how to start a *successful* career as a doula.

The top questions on the minds of most new doulas are:
Is there a demand for my kind of doula services?
How will I find clients?
When I find clients, how much can I charge?
Do I have to start my own business if I'm charging people?

Part 4 is going to answer all these questions and more!

Part 4

Preparing for a Doula Career

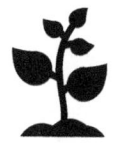

CHAPTER 17

Is There a Demand for Doulas?

It can be very reassuring to know there's demand for a job before getting trained for it. Unfortunately, you're not going to find job statistics for doulas, so you're going to have to be a bit more creative in finding this information. In this chapter, I'll show you how to research opportunities for your chosen doula role.

There are few factors you want to consider to determine demand for your field:

- Where you live
- The abundance of doulas in your area
- Who your ideal clients are
- The number of potential client situations in your area
- How well-known the problem is for your ideal clients

NOTE: If you plan to work virtually and not focus on a local market, some of these factors will not matter for you. However, marketing your services is much more challenging in a wider market, which you'll learn about in the section about marketing.

Here are the steps to research doula demand where you live:

Step 1:

Do internet research on the town/city where you live. To use a fishing analogy: where you live dictates the size of the pond you are fishing in and the kind of fish in that pond.

Consider the population of your town/city and its demographic makeup. How many adults, children, women, men, elderly, etc. live there? You can find this information at www.censusreporter.org. Just enter your town or city's name and you'll find data on population, number of people in each age group, marital status, birth rate, income, and more.

If you live in a community dominated by retired couples and you are a birth doula, you can see the challenge that might arise.

Step 2:

How many doulas are already in your area? Again, you're going to turn to the internet for this information. Enter "[type of] doula near me" in the search bar and see how many entries (or pages of entries) appear. For example, if I enter "divorce doulas near me," I see three Google business entries for *birth* doulas, and a list of search results for divorce doulas that don't live anywhere near me.

What does that tell me? There's room for my services as a divorce doula where I live. (Those results also tell me that I have to be very careful when I look at the results to see if they are what I asked for!)

And from my research in Step 1, I know that there are plenty of married people in my town. Yay! The downside: I may have to educate my community on the benefits of my type of doula, but otherwise, I'll be the one big fish in the pond.

But what if there are pages and pages of doulas that show up in your search result? Does that mean the market is already saturated with doulas? No. Just the opposite. If there are tons and tons of your type of doulas already in your area, that means that market has been *proven* for your field and is in demand.

You might have to do a bit more marketing to get yourself seen in a big pond of doulas, but you don't have to worry that people won't know what a doula is!

Step 3:

Do your ideal clients live near you?

This step has two parts to it. First, you have to identify your ideal clients. Your ideal client (or target market) is more than "pregnant people" for birth doulas. You want to get a bit more specific, like "pregnant teens" or "people pregnant with twins" or "transgender pregnant people." Or perhaps you want to work with someone of the same race or religion. You're going to learn more about identifying your ideal client in the marketing section, so for now, just know that you want to factor them into your research.

The second part is to determine if there are many of your ideal clients where you live. Is the internet going to tell you how many pregnant teens are near you? No, it's not. You're going to have to use your observation and intuition for this one. And again, the numbers alone don't dictate if there will be demand for you or not. If you are an immigrant who wants to work with other immigrants but there are few in your neighborhood, you could be in huge demand or have a hard time finding your ideal clients. If your work can be done virtually, casting a wider net to immigrant communities around your state or country could be a good solution. You can also choose to work with a wider demographic but specialize in working with your ideal clients.

I recently heard a story from a woman living with her enlisted husband on a military base. She was into organic gardening, herbal medicine, and home birth. She assumed she was the only "hippie chick" on the base because everyone else seemed so "conservative." When she became pregnant and found a local midwife, her midwife told her about all the other military parents in her care. She started a home birth community on her base, became a birth doula for military parents, and the rest is history. So who you are looking for could be right in your own backyard. Getting out and about, networking, and asking around may reveal just the folks you are looking for.

Step 4:

Is your doula field represented where you live?

If you are a healthcare or prison doula, are there hospitals or prisons in your community? Are abortions legal in the state where you live if you want to be an abortion doula? The absence of hospitals, prisons, or safe reproductive care does not mean you can't be that kind of doula. In fact, your role could be even more important for people having difficulty accessing those services. It does mean you may have to be open to travel or more creative ways of supporting clients.

You can do an internet search on the number of hospitals, adoption agencies, prisons, etc. in your area.

Step 5:

Do people in your area have a problem you can solve?

Marriage and divorce, birth and death, cancer and courtrooms are facts of life. Not everyone has a terrible experience in these types of life circumstances. But doulas can always make an experience better.

As doulas, we don't want to shine a light on problems people aren't aware of, and yet, we want people to know their options. Many people aren't aware they have a right to individualized care, emotional support, respect, or being listened to.

As a doula, you will become an ambassador for enhanced support in your field. You can hold information sessions that promote doula care, work with marginalized groups that are at higher risk of substandard care, speak at community events to raise awareness of gaps in the systems, and "create demand" if it doesn't exist already. All of this must be done ethically, of course, to not create fear and divisiveness.

Working within your community to elevate people's life experiences is the goal of a doula. When people have higher expectations, the demand for doulas increases.

CHAPTER 18

Marketing and Finding Clients

You've done your market research, and you know if you have a waiting population of clients or some education to do in your community. Now we're going to set your sights on the day-to-day tasks of being a doula.

A large part of working as a doula involves finding potential clients and getting hired. Once you get hired, you have to support your clients and manage the doula-client relationship. In most locales, you will also need to get a business license and do the tasks of running a business.

This chapter will focus on finding clients and getting hired. The next chapter will focus on starting and running your doula business.

Marketing 101

Finding clients is called "marketing" in business. Marketing sounds scary or distasteful to many people. I sure hated it when I started my business. But that's because I didn't know what marketing was. So let me set the record straight...

Marketing is the activity of promoting and selling products or services (that might sound kind of yucky to you). It's also the act of satisfying and retaining customers (now that doesn't sound so bad, does it?). Marketing gets people interested in your product or service (that sounds downright necessary!).

But most importantly, marketing is the process of identifying customer needs and determining how best to meet those needs. You have to know these things if you're going to be successful and happy in your work.

Marketing often gets confused with advertising, slimy salespeople, and numbers-crunching. But it's not that complicated. Advertising is simply *paying* to promote your business (which is just one part of marketing). There's nothing wrong with running paid ads if it helps you get great clients. And luckily, most doulas are not slimy people and couldn't do pushy marketing if they wanted to. And even more luckily, doulas don't usually have businesses that are large enough to warrant analysis and market research. Whew! You know how your business is doing because you see the results, talk with each of your clients one-on-one, and hear feedback directly.

Want to know the key to good marketing?

1. Identify your specific ideal client
2. Figure out the best way to reach them
3. Find out what problems they are experiencing
4. Explain how your services are the solution to their problems
5. Differentiate yourself from other doulas
6. Listen to what your clients want and fill that niche

Finding Clients

What ideas do you have for finding your first clients? You may have thought of posting on social media, hanging flyers at your church or community groups, putting an ad in Craigslist, or leaving business cards at a local coffee shop.

All of these are great ideas (and forms of marketing—see, you can be a marketer after all)! Basically, any idea you have is a great idea. Every channel you can think of to promote your doula work should be used.

When should you start looking for your first clients? Now!

You can start looking for clients before you are trained, and before you officially start your business. My advice is to start looking for them as soon as you are ready to talk to potential clients, because it can take awhile to get the word out.

The #1 way to build your doula clientele is by word of mouth. Tell everyone you know—everyone—that you are becoming a doula. Tell friends, relatives, co-workers, neighbors, folks at church, and people you meet in your community. The people you tell do NOT need to be your ideal clients. Everyone knows someone—or will eventually know someone—who will have a life situation in your field of work. People are much more likely to take the recommendation of someone they know than to go searching for a doula on their own. By the way, always have a few business cards to give to folks once you have piqued their interest.

Now that you've told everyone you know that you're a doula, it's time to reach out to people you don't know.

Your Ideal Client Avatar

At first, you may want any client that comes along. You want to put your new skills into practice and start changing lives! And that is great. But I'm going to encourage you (and later on insist) that you develop your *ideal client avatar.*

An ideal client avatar is the most important building block of your marketing efforts. We have a saying in marketing:

"If you're marketing to everyone, you're marketing to no one."

What that means is, if you aren't specific in who you are talking to or trying to reach, no one will pay attention. And that's because no one sees themselves as "generic," so you have to talk to your ideal client specifically.

Identifying your ideal client is one of the easiest parts of marketing. You're basically designing your *dream* client. How fun is that?! *Ask yourself: How old are they? Where do they live? Where do they shop? What are their hobbies, beliefs, or passions?* You could include their income, educational level, religions, politics, gender, or other demographics if that makes a difference to you or your work. But the most straightforward question to answer is: *Who would I most enjoy working with?* (Hint: Most doulas end up describing themselves, or who they were when they first had the problem they are trying to solve with their doula work.)

Don't worry that creating an ideal client avatar will limit you to only those clients. You will always reach a broader range of clients, but by targeting your ideal clients, you'll attract more of them to your work (and perhaps repel your *not* ideal clients in the process, which is a win-win).

So how do you attract your ideal clients? Here are three ways to do that:

1. Printed Materials

Business cards are an inexpensive way to promote your business locally. You can get cards made up that include your business name, maybe a logo, your phone number, and email address. Include your website if you have one. I know, I know...who uses business cards anymore? But business cards are great for leaving in your local coffee shop, or giving to all those people you told you're becoming a doula, or to people you meet out in public.

Note: Do not wait to get a perfect design, or to have a website, or to be certified, or any other excuse to not get some cards printed. You can get cards printed (and designed) for free from Vistaprint.com (you just pay for shipping). Only get a few hundred printed if you know you're going to change some of the information. Once they feel "perfect," pay to have them professionally printed.

You can also go to your local print shop—or use a home printer if you have one—to create a flyer. You'll only need a few flyers for places you go that have a bulletin board. Think churches, community centers, local grocery stores, schools. You only need one per bulletin board. You can get free designs online or from a platform like Canva. Start with your logo or the name of your business, a graphic element that will attract attention, a question that asks if the reader has this problem, a few bullet points that describe the benefits of your services, a mini bio, and how to contact you.

Here's an example:

Mending Hearts Divorce Doula Services

Are you going through a rough divorce and feel all alone?

A divorce doula can:

- » Help you navigate the legal and emotional process of divorce
- » Be by your side and advocate for your wishes
- » Help you with stress reduction
- » Be a compassionate listener

Deborah Jones has been serving the Seattle community for five years as a divorce doula. With her experience as a legal aide and her own journey through and beyond divorce, she has supported dozens of people through the emotional, logistical, financial, and legal challenges of ending a marriage.

To learn more about how I can help you, please visit my website at www.divorcedoula.com or call me at 555-111-2222 to schedule a free consultation.

Rack cards are a fancier option for promotional materials about your business. A rack card is a postcard-sized sheet that is a combination of a business card and a flyer. It can contain all the information on a flyer in a smaller size, and is often displayed in racks in offices or business spaces. Rack cards are more expensive to print than either business cards or a flyer because they are on heavier paper stock and often include multiple colors. For that reason, be very selective about where you place them, and only put them in places your *ideal* clients visit.

Those are my top suggestions for printed materials, and I want to stress that they are used only in hyper-local marketing (small towns, or your specific neighborhood or a targeted business in a larger city).

2. Digital Marketing

Digital marketing is a fancy word for "stuff on the internet." Websites, social media, and online ads are all forms of digital marketing.

The key piece of digital marketing that every business needs is a **website**. Having a website does not mean it's going to be a magnet to attract people to your business, or that people will even find your site by doing an internet search. That might happen, but most importantly, your website serves as an information hub—or landing spot—for people who have your website address and are looking you up.

You can create your own website on sites such as GoDaddy, Squarespace, or Wix. Use one of these user-friendly and inexpensive sites if you do not care about being found with internet searches. If you *do* want to be found by people who don't already have your website address, find a website designer or a DIY tool to help you build a WordPress site. That will provide the best SEO (search engine optimization) results for you.

Another way to get found or to promote your work is on **social media**. If you are a user of sites like Instagram, Facebook, TikTok, or LinkedIn, you may enjoy using social media to spread the word. Consider your ideal client and your field of work, and choose the social media platform that appeals most to that demographic.

You can make any type of post that speaks to your ideal client, showcases your work, educates viewers about your doula role, and reveals the behind-the-scenes life of a doula. Basically, anything that will educate or inform, engage, entertain, and promote to people who might be interested in your work as a doula.

Keep in mind that you don't control your social media platform and you don't own any of the content. Your platform may not let you link to your website. You could get locked out one day and lose all your contacts and everything you've ever posted. Social media limits your ability to reach everyone you want to with its ever-changing algorithms. So be mindful that even if you have one thousand followers, only three people may see your posts.

The good news is that social media is a great way to grow your audience, the people who are interested in what you are doing and "follow" you. You can set up a group to create a community of people with similar interests, with you and your work at the center. You can listen to what your followers are talking about, poll them, and support them. And then you can market and promote your services to them.

You can also **run ads** in online groups, Google ads, publications, blogs, listservs, intranets, or other online platforms. These are typically ads that you pay for that target certain audiences based on location, interests, employer, or industry. You could run ads directly for your clients, or to promote the doula role to other professionals in an industry that may be interested in partnering with you. There are also special sites that offer listing services that match clients seeking a doula to doulas who create a profile on the site.

Other forms of digital marketing include emails, texts, and videos, but those are usually not necessary for doulas in a local market.

3. Networking

A huge part of thriving as a doula is finding your community of professionals to collaborate with. You don't have to be an experienced or established doula to begin networking. Start looking in your local area now for other doulas, and for other professionals who work with your clients, to meet and learn about their work.

If you've been a client in the field you'll be working in, reach out to the professionals you worked with and tell them about your new business and how your services could benefit their clients. Ask them if they would like to be on your resource list of people you refer your clients to. Then ask if they would be willing to have some of your business or rack cards on hand to give to their clients.

If you don't have any personal connections with professionals in your industry, send a letter of introduction to a few professionals who have offices near you, letting them know you are a doula who is building a list of people to refer your clients to. Try to find some connection—they live on the same block, went to the same college, have kids in the same school as your kids. Ask if they'd like to be on your list, and if they would be willing to refer their clients to you.

Don't be hurt if someone you reach out to already has a doula they refer to. Most will be happy to add another one. And don't stop trying if you don't hear back from those first contacts. Just keep at it, and you will eventually have some new colleagues who will refer to you and appreciate your referrals to them in return.

Another great networking option is a local conference. Most industries have state or regional organizations that hold conferences. It's a great way to meet many people affiliated with your field of work and share about the benefits of doula support for their clients. You could even sponsor the conference or have an exhibitor table where you hand out materials, talk about your work, and collect business cards or contact information from conference attendees.

If being "on" like that is not your cup of tea, be sure to at least visit all the exhibitor tables, collect their business cards, ask about their work, tell them about yours, and see if any connections are made. Notice who you really liked, and who you'd like to get to know more. Then call or email them and see if you can build a relationship.

Networking is not a "do once and you're done" business activity. You have to regularly nurture your relationships, and build new ones. Add an hour of networking each week to your office calendar, reaching out to new professionals to network with and connecting with those already on your list. This will keep your incoming referrals, and referral list, growing.

The challenges of marketing

Marketing is relatively easy, once you can answer these three questions:

1. Who is your customer?
2. What are your customer's problems?
3. How do you help solve those problems?

The trick to marketing is being super clear about 1, 2, and 3 (most business owners aren't clear at all). Then all you have to do is find a way to explain those things quickly to people with a short attention span.

There is no instinct or intuitive knowing hardwired into human nature that tells us how to run a business or market our services. But some of the components of business management and marketing are intuitive: how to connect with other people, how to communicate effectively, and understanding what motivates people into action.

The best way to connect with others is through empathy—having a shared understanding of another. I bet you, the doula, already have an innate understanding of what your potential clients are struggling with. You can use your empathy to connect with them around their "problem." That is the root of marketing.

Selling yourself and your services relies on compassionate communication—being honest about who you are, sharing your unbridled passion, pointing out your personal strengths, and using non-jargony words to describe your work.

Empathy and compassionate communication are going to be your most valuable marketing skills.

But you can't market once and be done. You have to keep at it. Keep updating your website, replenish your business and rack cards around town, reach out to other professionals once a week, and nurture the networking relationships you already have.

You can tell when you have done a good job promoting your business: you will get inquiry calls at a steady pace in the volume you desire, you will be getting calls from the right clients, you will get hired at least 50 percent of the time, and you will love the clients you are working with. Each of these things means you marketed in the right place, to the right people, at the right time, and you said the right thing to make them contact you.

That is how fun good marketing can be, and it feels as good as chocolate mousse tastes when it is working well.

Interviewing Potential Clients

Once you have attracted your ideal clients, you finally get to talk to them! The idea of meeting a potential client face-to-face can be exciting, scary, and welcome all at once. Once you get the hang of doing them, I hope they become fun.

Doulas typically schedule an interview or "meet and greet," an informal face-to-face meeting with the client(s). This visit is an opportunity for you and the clients to see how you feel being around each other, because choosing a doula is not like choosing a stockbroker. While someone definitely wants to trust their stockbroker with their finances, they don't usually expect to form an emotional bond with them. Not so with a doula.

Because the doula role is inherently more personal and emotion-based, the interview is a *two-way interview*. You want to see if you want to work with this client as much as they are deciding if they want to work with you. You'll get to learn more about what kind of support your client is looking for, and they'll get more details on how you work as a doula and what your services include.

The meeting should be free and no obligation to the client. Plan on about forty-five minutes, and make sure anyone you'll be working for will attend (for example, if you are a birth doula interviewing a client who is in a couple, you'll want both partners to be present).

After the pandemic when people got used to Zoom, they either never want to leave their homes or never want to step foot on Zoom again. So you might offer the option of in-person or virtual meetings for your clients. Or, if *you* have a preference, you can set them up the way you like.

Some doulas or clients will prefer to meet in person so they can see what it feels like to be in that person's presence. But most people can get that sense even over Zoom. Keep in mind that if you meet in person, you (and your clients) will have to travel, which costs time and money. Or, you can save them the hassle and offer to meet at their home if you are comfortable with that.

I advise setting up a free scheduling system like Calendly, where you can set your availability and clients can select a date and time to meet. All you have to do is send clients a link. Nothing sucks time like trying to schedule something with back-and-forth emails. Having set times for your interview will protect your schedule and your sanity!

Once the interview is scheduled, prepare yourself to answer common questions that potential clients will have. For most doula roles, that will include:

- How long have you been doing this?
- How many clients have you served? How many clients do you take at once?
- What kind of experience do you have with [people in my situation]?
- What do your services include?

- Do you coach us from afar or attend with us in person?
- How do you help us cope with challenging situations?
- When can we reach you? How do we reach you? What if we can't reach you?
- What are your fees? When do you get paid?
- What if we aren't satisfied with something? How do we address that?
- Do you offer discounts?

The specific questions will vary based on the type of doula, but you get the idea. Be prepared to answer these questions. A good trick is to write down your answers to every question you think of, read them out loud, and then have a friend "interview" you so you can practice responding in the moment. Another important note: If your clients don't know what questions to ask, have a spiel ready to provide important information. And never leave an interview without talking about your fees!

As the interview closes, you will let the clients know what to expect next. Can they hire you on the spot? Will you send them your contract to review before making a decision? Do you want them to decide within a certain time frame (maybe you have other clients waiting to interview you if you don't get hired)? Agree on a date by which you'll hear back from them, and send them a nice follow-up email or text after the interview.

You can learn a lot more about interviewing techniques in one of my online courses or business workbooks, or you can get my fabulous client attraction, interview script, and closing technique formula in *The Doula Success Formula*. Visit my website at www.carriekenner.com for details.

Getting hired

If you haven't heard from a client by the appointed date, don't hesitate to follow up with them. Just politely ask if they've made a decision or need a bit more time. If you don't feel compelled to work with them, you could also use this opportunity to let them know you are no longer available and offer referrals to other doulas.

But if they want to hire you, yay! (Congratulations, by the way.) It's time to initiate the "onboarding" process. You'll have your client(s) sign your contract and pay a deposit to reserve your services. You should always, always have a contract in place, even if you are taking a client free of charge. Contracts don't enforce payment; they clarify agreements and set mutual expectations. You can find sample contracts in my business workbook, with any of my business courses, or by doing an internet search.

From there, you'll likely have intake forms for your clients to complete and your first meeting to schedule. You also might have an internal process for yourself to keep track of your clients, send information, schedule visits, and request payments. Get all those beginning pieces in place so you have everything ready to go.

In the next chapter, I'll talk about how to manage your clients through the entire process of working with you. Your process might be fully automated with a client management system that sends things automatically according to a preset schedule, or you can go a simpler route and have online forms that you send a link to access.

> Planning to make being a doula your new career? Check out my business and marketing courses, guides, workbooks, and business coaching program at doula-training.carriekenner.com

CHAPTER 19

Business Basics

If you plan to earn money as a doula, you will likely need a business license in your city, county, and/or state. Most doulas are caught off guard when they find out they have to open a business. Don't worry if you know nothing about running a business (or if the thought of it makes you panic). It's easier than you think, and I'm going to outline the basic steps here so you know what to expect.

In this chapter, I'll show you how to do your own research on business structures, professional requirements, finances, liabilities, and where to find more answers. You'll also learn about different business models to choose from, how to track income and expenses, how to set your fees, and how to maintain business records.

And if having a business completely freaks you out, you can work for an agency if they exist in your community (or take my JumpStart Your Doula Business program, where I walk you through all the steps to start and manage your doula business). Knowing this process will give you the confidence, inspiration, and motivation to keep going and not let starting a business derail your doula career.

In a nutshell, here's what you have to do to open and run your own business:

1. Get a business license and business bank account
2. Get any required registrations, certifications, or insurance
3. Track income and expenses
4. Manage your clients
5. Maintain business records

Starting a Doula Business

There are some "official" things you will do to start your business, and some operational (day-to-day) things. The first "official" act is getting a business license. The second is setting up a business bank account. But first, you need to know the kind of business *model* you will use, as that will dictate the type of business *structure* you will form.

Different Business Models

There are many business models you can operate under as a doula. You can work as a doula on your own, with a partner, as part of a collective, for a doula agency, or for an organization or facility that employs doulas.

Most doulas work independently as a **sole proprietor.** This is the simplest and quickest way to get started. You get your own clients, set up your own systems, and make it up as you go.

Working with a **partner** or as part of a **collective** can be enjoyable and rewarding, but requires much more communication, planning, and coordination. You can't fly by the seat of your pants if another person is involved. And for all the extra work of coordinating and communicating with your partner/s…you have to share the income. Partnerships and collectives are definitely a good option, but think very seriously about what you are getting into, especially as you are starting out.

The most successful partnerships and collectives that I have seen are started by experienced doulas. Those doulas know the ropes, know their style, know what they like to do and what they don't, and know what they are looking for in a partner or group. They can explain their needs, strengths, and weaknesses, and that leads to a stronger collaboration than if two or more new doulas are trying to figure out how to work together as they go .

Working for a **doula agency** is a great way to get started if you don't want to run your own business. The agency does all the work of finding clients and handling the finances; you work directly with the clients and get paid by the agency, usually as an independent contractor. You may still need to get a business license, because many organizations require you to be a legal business entity that they contract with. You will be responsible for your own business expenses and will want to deduct them from your taxes.

The downside of working for an agency? They typically keep one-third or more of the doula fee the client pays. The trade-off may be worth it to you. Or working for an agency might be a great way to start, until you get some experience and are ready to go off on your own.

There are only a handful of opportunities to **get hired by a facility**—such as a hospital—in the United States. Some hospitals have birth or death doula programs that contract with doulas to serve their patients; even fewer hire doulas as staff members. There are dozens of community-based organizations (usually non-profits) that hire or contract with different kinds of doulas to serve their clientele, and hundreds of doula agencies that find the clients and have a group of contracted doulas that serve them.

If you find a program that hires doulas, the benefit of being an employee is that you have a set income and (hopefully) benefits. The downside is that you may not get to choose your clients, or work with them from start to finish like an independent doula does. As you learn more about your doula role, you will take these differences into account when deciding what kind of doula practice you'd like to have.

Whatever business model you decide on when you start, know that you can change it in the future.

Business Structures

There are a few business *structures* to choose from in the United States (and similar options in other countries): sole proprietor, limited liability corporation (or partnership), nonprofit, or S-corporation. Each structure has its pros and cons, so you need to choose the one that will work best for you. Here is a summary of the features of each; be sure to research each one more fully by visiting your state's business licensing department or website:

Sole Proprietor This is the most common, the easiest, and the cheapest business license to obtain. With this license, you and your business are a single entity. The license is filed under your social security number, and your income from this business is filed with your personal federal income tax form.

Pros: Cheapest of all the business licenses to obtain. Get it once and it's good for life.

Cons: If you are sued, your personal assets could be at risk, since you and your business are the same.

Limited Liability Corporation (LLC) or Partnership This is the second most common business structure for doulas. It's a bit more complicated to obtain, and more expensive. With this license, you and your business are separate entities. It will still be created with your social security number, but you can get a separate tax ID number (or Federal Employer Identification Number) as well. Your income from this business can also be filed with your federal personal income tax, OR you can request to file it as a separate entity.

Pros: If you are sued, your personal assets are more protected, and only assets from your business are at risk. You may be able to file your taxes separately from your personal taxes, which could result in tax benefits. Consult with a tax advisor on this.

Cons: More complicated forms to fill out. More expensive license to obtain. Limited liability companies must file an annual report to the Secretary of State.

Non-Profit This is the second least common type of business license for doulas. It is much more complex to obtain (you have to qualify to be a non-profit), but has significant tax benefits, so may be worth it if you are going to function as a non-profit organization.

Pros: If you are sued, your personal assets are protected, and only assets from your business are at risk. Non-profit organizations enjoy significant tax breaks.

S-Corporation This is the least common type of business license for doulas. It is more complex to obtain, but may offer significant tax benefits. An S-corp is similar to a limited liability company in that the owner(s) and business are separate entities. S-corp taxes are paid separately from individual taxes, and profits and losses are "passed through" to owners.

Pros: If you are sued, your personal assets are protected, and only assets from your business are at risk. You can pay yourself a "salary." Tax rates may be lower for the business than self-employment taxes. Consult with a tax advisor on this.

Cons: More complicated paperwork to file. More expensive license to obtain. You may need to file an annual report to the Secretary of State.

I hope your head isn't swimming in confusion right now. It can all seem very foreign if owning a business is brand new to you. But it can be learned. My recommendation is to start with the easiest structure first, and change it if the need arises. Your business will evolve over time, and you can always change your business structure.

Choose a Name for Your Business

Now, the fun part: Pick a name for your business. It could be your own name, like Carrie's Doula Services. Or it could be a catchy name, like Big Belly Services (my former business name). The trend for business names today is to just use your first and last name.

You will likely want to choose a name that is meaningful or soulful that speaks to you (and hopefully potential clients). Naming your business often feels as important as naming a child. But, trust me, it's not. Your clients are *not* going to hire you based on your business name. Sure, your name may stand out and attract people, but they are going to hire you based on *you*.

Before you confirm your business name, do an internet search and a trade name search (via your state's business licensing entity) to make sure no one else is using that name.

Next, get a business email address that includes your business name. Do not use your personal email address, especially if it's the same account you've had since high school! Your email address could be something like mydoulabusiness@gmail.com (free) or carrie@mywebsitename.com if you have a website. You want to keep your business mail separate from your personal mail, and you want to give this email address to all the entities you set up for your business (such as your bank account, which is next).

Get a Business License

Okay, you've decided on your business model and business structure, you've got a name for your business, and a new email address. Finally, you are ready to get your business license!

A business license is almost always required by your state, and may also be required by your city or county. You can find this information by looking up "Business license <your state>" on the internet, and start reading or call the office.

In the United States, your state's Department of Licensing (this is usually the agency that issues business licenses) will most likely let you know what other licenses you may need.

You can usually apply for a business license online, register your business name, and pay the fees. A few weeks later, you'll get a paper business license in the mail.

I recommend you get your license sooner rather than later because once you are an official business, any money you spend to start your business is an expense that you can deduct from next year's taxes.

Open a Business Bank Account

Now that you are an official business, you can get an official business bank account. Having a separate account for your business finances will make your life so much easier. All your income will go into this account, and all expenses will be purchased from it. You'll pay yourself from this account by writing yourself a check or transferring money to your personal account. It will be very easy to track income and expenses for your business this way.

The bank will need your business identification number and/or social security number to open your account. As with any bank account, there may be a monthly fee if you don't maintain a minimum balance, and business accounts usually have similar fees for other services such as overdrafts, stop check, or ATMs.

If you already have a personal bank account, you may want to use the same bank. I advise you to shop around for a no-fee account, one that has good terms or reward programs, and one that offers the conveniences you desire.

Professional Licenses, Regulations, and Certification

Professional licenses are different from business licenses. **Professional licenses** are granted by states to allow someone to provide a professional service—such as midwives, funeral directors, massage therapists, social workers, even electricians. Doulas typically do not need a license, as they are not performing a licensed level of service.

States also require some professionals to be **certified**. Two examples are substance-use counselors or nursing assistants. This **state certification** differs from doula certification offered by doula training organizations and is not required to work as a doula.

State licenses and certifications are required to *legally* practice in a field. **Doulas are not required by law** to be licensed or certified in any state or province at the time of this writing (2024). There have been a few cases where jurisdictions (states or facilities) have tried to challenge that but have failed. It is your responsibility to do an internet search for your doula role and region, and to contact any local doulas for updates.

You may also hear about **professional standards** or **protocols**. Protocols are practices or procedures that are put in place by an advisory board or collection of professionals to guide decision-making and safe actions within their field.

Doula organizations that certify doulas may have professional standards or a scope of practice that they expect their certified doulas to follow. These are optional for non-certified doulas. Doulas do not typically have protocols to follow.

It is important to understand that standards and protocols are not laws. Professionals who do not follow accepted standards or protocols may be banned, fined, or reprimanded within their industry, but they will not face legal action unless they are sued for those actions.

Liability Insurance

All this talk of laws, certification, and being sued may make you wonder if you will need **liability insurance** as a doula. Liability insurance is insurance that a business gets to cover them if they cause or get sued for damages, injury, or harm to a client. Clients could also sue for refunds or financial claims.

Most doula roles should inherently be protected for liability because doulas don't advise clients, perform clinical or legal tasks, or guarantee certain outcomes. But the reality is that anyone can sue anyone for anything, and doulas are no exception.

Doulas are not required by law to have liability insurance. However, if you work for a doula collective, agency, or program that contracts with doulas, they may require you to carry your own insurance.

There are many insurance companies that provide general liability insurance for businesses. If a client visited you in your home and fell, you would be covered for their injuries (this is one reason I don't recommend you have clients come to your home). If you broke a client's prized vase while in their home, your insurance would cover its value. If someone claimed you didn't show up to their event and sued you for irreparable emotional damage, your legal fees and any settlement would be covered.

Because the doula role is unique and often misunderstood, insurance companies may put you in the same category as licensed health care or legal providers. But since you don't have the credentials or license for that, they can't insure you. A bit of a catch-22.

Many doulas practice without insurance. Others don't feel comfortable with that risk and find some type of insurance. Others feel partially protected by having a limited liability company; at least they won't lose their home or other assets if they are sued.

There's no way to completely protect yourself from the threat of being sued. You get to decide for yourself if you are prepared to face that situation if it occurs, or if the risk of being sued warrants carrying insurance.

Setting Fees

Let's talk about something more pleasant—getting paid for your important work!

The fee you charge as a doula can vary greatly, depending on where you live, your level of experience, and other skills you have that are applicable to your doula work. If you are able to volunteer services or offer discounts, that is fine but not required. Do what makes you feel well-compensated for your work.

As you are starting out, do some research to see what other doulas are charging in your area. Do an online search and look at local doulas' websites. Many doulas will include their rates on their services page. If there are no other doulas in your area, pick a comparable town (region, size, and economy) and see what doulas there are offering.

Many doulas don't feel comfortable charging anything—or much—when they are first starting out. They feel uncertain and don't want to get paid until they feel more experienced. This is not necessary, as we know that the presence of a trained person improves experiences and outcomes for clients no matter how experienced they are.

Be careful to not confuse "experience" with "always knowing what to do." After attending hundreds of births, I still never knew exactly what I was going to do when I stepped into someone's birth space! So if you've worked with a few clients and are thinking, "Hey, I'm learning a lot and really adding value for these folks," or "I really love what I'm doing but I don't think I can keep doing this for free/such low cost," then start charging or charging more.

It may be easier to get your first clients if you offer your services at a lower rate than experienced doulas, but it may also depend on your field and expertise. Do be mindful of what more experienced doulas are charging in your area and price yourself respectfully. Overcharging (which makes doula services inaccessible to the average person), as well as undercharging (which makes it impossible for doulas to survive), can devalue the work of doulas everywhere.

If you are working for an agency or organization, your rates may be dictated for you. If you are working for yourself, you can raise your rates as you see fit.

Like any career, you hopefully intend to grow. Whether it is adding additional skills over time, raising your rates, or adding packaged services, you are in the driver's seat.

Doulas often raise their rates every five, ten, or twenty clients when they are starting out, because their learning curve is exponential. This is one of the perks—and responsibilities—of owning your own business! **When you feel**

appropriately compensated for your time, skills, and service, you will be able to continue doing this work without resentment or burnout.

Tracking Income and Expenses

Once you are an official business, start to track your income and expenses. Income is simply what people pay you (your fee plus tips, or the value of a gift or trade). Expenses are anything you buy or pay for to operate your business, such as supplies in your office, a laptop for your business, gas and mileage to visit clients, your cell phone bill, parking fees, and more.

Keep receipts of all income and expenses and enter the date, amount, and source in a spreadsheet, or even just a notebook, so it's all in one place for compiling and reporting later. This will make filing state and federal income taxes a breeze (versus a tornado).

You can find sample finance tracking sheets in my business courses and workbooks at www.carriekenner.com, or online. You can get as fancy as getting software like QuickBooks, or as simply as creating an Excel or Google spreadsheet. The tracking system is not the key; regularly entering income and expenses is.

As I mentioned before, you cannot deduct expenses until you are a business entity, so get your business license before you start buying stuff. Even if you get a quick-and-easy sole proprietor license, you can now start tracking expenses that you can deduct at tax time. They really make a difference, especially in your first years of business.

Managing Clients

You are a business and now you are getting clients. To make your business easy to manage, you want to set up a system to manage clients from beginning to end.

You can start by writing out all the interactions you'll have with your clients:

- first contact
- interview
- onboarding (signing the contract, collecting the deposit, getting initial forms)
- scheduling visits
- sending information
- attending visits
- attending events (birth, abortion, surgery, death, etc.)
- follow-up after the event
- collecting payments
- closing the relationship

There may be other steps along the way you want to keep track of. You can set up your client management system however you like.

You may find pre-packaged client management systems, such as Honeybook, Dubsado, or ClickUp. They may be more complicated to set up, have more features than you need, and be more costly than you want, but check them out to see if they could be a helpful tool for you.

You can also create a spreadsheet or paper tracking sheet with your client's names down the left-hand column and the important tasks listed across the top. Just check off each task when it's completed, and you'll be able to see at a glance what needs to be done next for each client.

When you have multiple clients, it will get confusing. As you are working with your first clients, notice what will help you when you have a bunch of them. If you are out and about a lot, think about something you can access from your phone. If you're an office-based person, that may not matter as much.

When you have completed your work with a client, consider how you will close the relationship. A sense of completion will be helpful for you and your clients; it's one of the key steps in the process of transformation!

Closing the relationship often consists of a final visit to debrief and process their experience. You may have a small closing ritual to acknowledge what they have been through and the work you have done together. You can offer a small "parting gift" such as a journal, photo, quote, self-care product, or treat. This is entirely optional! And don't be surprised if they have a gift for you.

Maintain business records

Taking Notes

Whenever you communicate with your clients, you will need to keep notes on what was discussed, decisions that were made, and action steps for you or your clients. You will need to know which topics you covered already, your clients' priorities, and topics you want to discuss further.

The purpose of your notes is to be able to refer to them in the future—before the next visit, before you join them in person, or if they are calling you in a few years to review something.

It is not reassuring to your clients for you to ask them the same questions repeatedly, or to appear not to remember what they said they wanted; that does not build trust.

At first, you may think you'll remember everything; you'll be hanging on to their every word and not forget a thing. And maybe you will when you only have one or two clients. But as you have more clients, more details, and more stories piling up—or you simply don't have a great memory—you will not remember the specifics of individual visits or calls.

There are two ways to take notes: you can either take notes during the conversation—whether remotely or in person—or capture them when you're done.

It takes a bit of technique to take notes in an unobtrusive way *during* an in-person visit. Here's how to start:

- Practice jotting down notes on a notepad (paper or electronic) as you ask questions and listen intently (it's tricky but not impossible).
- DO pay more attention to your clients than your notes.
- Jot down a word or two to remind you of something you want to come back to later.
- DO ask for a pause if you need to catch up on your notes for a moment before moving on.

If you don't like taking notes during a conversation, allow time after a visit or discussion to capture the highlights of the conversation. I used to do this in my car after a visit before driving home. The topics were fresh in my mind, and writing them down helped cement them in my memory. I could also identify any topics I wanted to follow up on.

The notes you'll be taking aren't legal records or part of a medical chart, so they don't have to be written in a certain way. You'll probably develop your own system of note-taking and abbreviations as you go.

Note: Recording a conversation is not typically done. It may not feel safe to clients and appears overly formal.

Record Keeping

For every client, you will need to maintain records about your work together. This will include notes from all your visits, as well as other documents related to your client. Here are the typical documents you will have for each client:

- Intake form
- Signed contract
- Notes from pre-event visits or phone calls
- All text, email, or other app-supported communication

- Notes from the event, if you attended with them
- Notes from follow-up visits
- You may also maintain a library of common resources you share with clients, samples or templates, links to articles, referral lists, and other handouts.

You may keep client information using electronic files, digital documents, or paper records as long as they are in a locked place. If you use paper files, you must store them in a locked briefcase, file cabinet, or closet. If you use digital files, they must be in a password protected folder or device. If you use an electronic records system, your account must be password protected. All files sent electronically must use an encrypted email system or software. Your field may also have specific requirements for keeping client records.

Most doulas aren't required to maintain client records, or keep them for a set period of time. We do this voluntarily and to help us provide excellent services. I kept my "active" client files with me at all times (I was an on-call doula). Once I had my final visit with clients, I "closed" their file and put it in a safe place for long-term storage. You may destroy your client files after a period of time, or archive them.

CHAPTER 20

Community and Family Support

If you will be working in a doula role that requires you to be on call or work in high-stress situations such as courtrooms, prisons, cancer care, or end-of-life, you will need the emotional support of your family and friends, and a supportive community of like-minded doulas.

Community Support

The number one cause of doula burnout is isolation. Therefore, the number one tool for a long-term career is community.

A huge part of thriving as a doula is finding a community of colleagues. You don't have to be an experienced or established doula to begin. Start looking in your local area, in online groups, or on social media for other doulas or professionals working in your field in a caring, compassionate way.

Join these groups, reach out to individuals that you feel aligned with, and ask to meet one-on-one if necessary. Pay attention and access the resources they share for continuing education, connection, and collaboration. Nurture those relationships with meet-ups, coffee dates, or Zoom chat sessions.

You can also develop debriefing relationships with your colleagues. There may be situations where you need a compassionate ear to listen to how you handled a case, discuss a difficult client, ask for feedback, seek guidance, or just have a shoulder to cry on. It is important to set guidelines and boundaries for debriefing sessions; ask consent before you begin, let your listener know what kind of response you desire (just listening, empathy, reflection, or suggestions, etc.), and expect absolute confidentiality in what is shared.

Having a number of doula colleagues can make all the difference in your sense of community and confidence as a doula.

Family and Friends Support

Many doulas discover that their newfound doula skills and passion spill over into their personal lives as well. This can be met with curiosity, befuddlement, or resistance by their friends and family members. It is normal for humans to be concerned when someone in their inner circle changes. Change represents growth, and to be honest, growth can be hard. So give your family and friends grace if they start to question your new doula role.

At the same time, you must request grace and patience from them. You *will* be changing, and it can sometimes be messy. It may take you a few months to get comfortable in your doula role, and to pass that *"Oh my god I must tell everyone what it's like being a doula!"* phase.

If you are working in a doula role that requires being on call or schedule flexibility, you may no longer be as available to your family and friends. Take the time to explain *why* you have to be on call (some events like birth and death are unpredictable, other events arise urgently, like a suddenly rescheduled surgery). And explore with them *how* to manage being on call.

When I was a full-time birth doula, I had four clients every month. All of my prenatal and postpartum visits with those clients were scheduled, but I knew that four times during the month, I was going to get a call that my client was in labor and I needed to join them.

The truth of being on call is that you don't get a phone call out of the blue and have to drop everything you are doing and rush to the hospital. That only happens on TV. The reality is that you may get numerous texts or "advance warning" calls—sometimes for days—before you actually need to go. Only once in my fifteen-year career did I have to go meet my clients at the first phone call.

But at some point, you do need to go, regardless of whatever is going on in your life. My ex-husband and I developed plans for 1) what to do if it was morning, before he went to work, 2) what to do if it was the middle of the day and he'd need to pick up our son, 3) what to do if it was evening or the middle of the night and he was home but would need to go to work in the morning. Keep in mind, we didn't have to figure this out in a moment's notice. But once those advance warnings started coming, we'd look at our calendars and work out a few plans for the coming days.

If he had meetings or obligations he couldn't cancel, we'd work on childcare options. If he was out of town, we'd have more elaborate plans. The point is, whatever responsibilities you have in your life—kids, pets, plants, elders, etc.—you need to have plans in place.

One thing that became part of my life was letting people know that, when I scheduled a meeting or appointment with them, I would be there "unless I was at a birth." That meant that I had to find doctors, dentists, massage therapists, and chiropractors that would not charge me a cancellation fee if I didn't notify them at least twenty-four hours before an appointment. The babies I worked with didn't give *me* twenty-four hours notice, so I had to pass on that inconvenience. Once I explained my situation to a care provider, they understood and wanted to support my work and agreed. If they didn't, I wouldn't work with them.

At first, it all sounds so exciting. Your family and friends will enthusiastically support your incredible work as a doula. They love the idea of championing the important work you are doing in the world. But the first time you miss your best friend's birthday party, an anniversary with your partner, or your own kid's graduation, you feel like shit and they feel betrayed. So be sure to get a backup doula for events you absolutely do not want to miss.

On the other end of being on call is the recovery, both physical and emotional. If you've attended a prolonged death, sat through a long miscarriage, endured a courtroom battle, or stayed at the bedside of your client with post-surgery complications, you may not arrive home with the capacity to dive right back into life. Over time, you will develop rituals and practices to protect your energy and your transitions in and out of work. Discussing your needs with those closest to you will help make those transitions as smooth as possible for all.

It is not uncommon for a doula's closest-in people to also be their sounding boards. Debriefing a challenging situation, venting about a shitty care provider, railing against an unjust system, and crying over a loss is something that most doula partners and friends get used to hearing. It is important to ask permission before you vent, and to request total confidentiality (they cannot repeat your feelings or stories to anyone else). They can also decide that "doula talk" is off limits with them. Respect their choices, as you can always find someone else willing to listen.

If your friends and family are willing listeners, let them set some boundaries on what (or how much) they are willing to take or not. You don't want to pass on the vicarious trauma (a negative reaction when someone is exposed to trauma through their work, or through hearing someone's story of trauma) that some doulas experience. Be respectful of their capacity to hold hard stories, and mindful of if your doula tales are dominating the time you spend together.

As you can see, being a doula has the potential to impact one's family and social circle both positively and negatively. Open communication is the key. Working out mutually-beneficial solutions is critical. And if an on-call or emotionally-charged lifestyle proves to be too much for you or your family, you now know about many other doula roles that may be a better fit.

CHAPTER 21

Ongoing Coaching and Doula Communities

One of the things I've noticed in my years of running businesses and coaching business owners is that it takes a good year to figure out what your business will be like. It will not be what you expected; some parts will be better than you hoped for, others will suck. But over time, you will determine what parts of your work you absolutely love, where you want to grow and expand, and what you'd like to throw off a cliff.

As your business and income grow, look for areas you can outsource to an assistant (or friend or family member who wants to support you). Do you need someone to set up your client management system? Do you want someone to schedule your social media or blog posts? Do you want to stop doing placenta encapsulations but would love a small referral fee for sending yours to another doula?

But if you can't even envision getting to the one-year mark, you might benefit from business coaching. I offer a nine-month group coaching program called *JumpStart Your Doula Career* that guides doulas through every step of setting up their business, getting their first clients, marketing, interviewing, onboarding, setting up business systems, finances, and so much more. It's a class and a community all in one.

Speaking of community, finding a doula community can be crucial to your career. There's nothing like having colleagues who truly understand what you do. They know the challenges of your field, what it's like to have your role misunderstood, and the trials of being a small-business owner. You can commiserate, collaborate, and celebrate together!

If a doula group doesn't exist in your community or for your field, start one! There are no rules on who can start a support group, or what you do in your group. Reach out to other doulas in your industry and suggest you start meeting on a regular basis. You can make it up as you go.

Becoming wise about business and your practice is the reward that comes from having run a business for a while. Most doulas start doing every facet of their business themselves—mainly because they can't afford or justify hiring anyone to do it for them—and then hone in on their specialties and strengths over the years.

You can fine-tune your business in terms of the services you provide (adding new ones or subtracting ones you don't enjoy), or how your business is managed (financial tracking, client management, marketing, taxes, etc.).

You can collaborate on service packages with other doulas in your community, outsource tasks to a virtual assistant, buy software to automate your systems, and hire professionals to take over your books.

Enjoy the wisdom that comes from experience, and the permission you can grant yourself to create a business you love with boundaries that keep it sustainable.

CLOSING

Is the Doula Lifestyle for You?

Becoming a doula will cause ripple effects within you, your family, your social life, your day-to-day routine, and how you see the world.

Something inside is hinting to you that being a doula is a big deal. You know it is more than just being fascinated by menstruation, or wanting to be around babies, or being passionate about justice. The ancient heart of you—the DNA of your ancestors circulating in your blood—whispers that you can be of great service if you walk down this path. Perhaps your pulse quickens, or the butterflies are dancing in your belly when you think about being a doula. Maybe adrenaline starts surging and you get scared. Or finally, you feel totally alive!

Whatever your body's response to the idea of being a doula, it is signaling to you that your life is about to change. What is your body trying to tell you? Perhaps that being a doula is sacred, unpredictable, and amazing.

As humans, we innately know that deeply supporting someone is profound—even though modern cultures have tried to downplay the power of human connection, authenticity, and compassion. Your inner self knows that you are embarking on a path that will change people's lives and lead to a better world, perhaps as your j.o.b.

Only you know if being a doula will fit into your life now or in the future. Using all the experiences you have amassed, consider if this is the time to embrace this work or if it should wait. You may need to have conversations with your family and community to gather their input and support. You will definitely need to make arrangements in various aspects of your life to support the lifestyle of a doula. Reflect back on all the ways in which you have evolved in your life so far; the rest of your life will be no different. If you decide being a doula is not feasible now, that doesn't mean it never will be!

If you are still unclear about your doula path after reading the solutions in this book, use all your creative genius, passion, and resourcefulness to overcome the obstacles you see in your way. If you need help sorting out your options, please reach out for support at www.doula-training.carriekenner.com.

"Unless someone like you cares a whole awful lot, nothing is going to get better. It's not."

—Dr. Seuss, *The Lorax*

ACKNOWLEDGMENTS

When I started writing my first book four years ago, I had no idea what I was stepping into. I thought I'd sit down for a few weeks or months, release onto the page all the information that was stored in my brain, find a publisher, and—voilà!—I'd be a published author.

If you've written a book, you can stop chuckling now.

Ask any experienced writer, and they'll tell you that no one writes a good book on their own. So let me thank the people who have helped make me a better writer and this a better book:

My first writing coaches: Cami Ostman and Dana Tye Rally

My editor who appeared at just the right time: Callie Stoker-Graham

My early readers and reviewers: Makeda Akoma, Sarafina Farwell, Heather Geiser, Fiore Grey, Jennifer Hirayama, Margaret Howieson, Veronica Malki, Erika Primozich, Nikki Shaheed, Lisa Tankersley, Tionni Townsend, and Stephanie Ziegers

My early mentors: Pam England, Penny Simkin, and Sandy Szalay

My old doula colleagues who taught me so much about how to be a great doula, particularly: Alissa Wehrman, Debra Shelden, Andrea Nesheim, Amy Kastelin, and Rebecca Shepherd

My doula students who always inspire me to be the best trainer ever

But nothing would make any sense, be worth it, or have any purpose if it wasn't for my family. Thank you to my three sons, Malik, Rahsaan, and Jacob for making me a mom and the person I am today. Thank you to my grandkids—De'Ja, Amajhé, Jaisaan, Tionni, Malia, Tyrell, Cadence, London, and Grayson—for being such amazing people who delight me to no end. And for the next generation of our family—Micah, Éla, Mila, January 2025 baby, and who else is to come—the work I do is for you. May life be a whole lot better when you're grown.

ABOUT THE AUTHOR

Carrie Kenner, BA, CD, is a writer, book-writing coach, renowned doula trainer, and business coach living in Washington state. Carrie was a birth doula and doula trainer for 20 years, and has trained over 2,500 doulas nationally and internationally. As a business coach and mentor, she has helped hundreds of doulas launch successful careers that have served tens of thousands of individuals and families.

Carrie has had many jobs in her life. But it wasn't until she became a doula that she found her *career*. Her most rewarding and impactful work has been as a birth doula to hundreds of families, and a doula trainer to thousands of doulas.

Carrie became a mom at 19. She gave birth at home, in her own bed, surrounded by five midwives, her partner, her mom, her partner's mom and little sister, and her best friend. At that moment, she didn't know a seed was being planted in her heart that would grow into the work that she would become known for. And it took a while for that seed to find the light of day…

While putting herself through college as a single mom of two boys, working her way up the corporate ladder in healthcare administration, buying a home and paying bills, and feeding her creative soul with pottery, painting, or playing piano, she dreamed of providing the exquisite care to others that her midwives provided to her. But midwifery school was expensive and she could barely afford the bills and to feed her sons.

Twenty years later, while pregnant with her third baby, she heard the word *doula*, and the seed finally sprouted. When she was eight months pregnant, she was laid off from her corporate job. Instead of trying to find another job that she wouldn't start until after maternity leave, she decided to fulfill her dream: she accepted a severance package and became a doula.

Carrie started Big Belly Services in 2001 in the basement of her Seattle, WA, home four months after her baby was born. With her son sleeping on her chest, she developed a website, printed brochures, and made phone calls. Her sole proprietor business offered Birthing From Within childbirth education classes and birth doula services. Two years later, she formed an LLC, hired an office assistant, and brought on new instructors. The following year, she added local and national doula trainings, conference presentations, advanced doula workshops, business coaching, and retreats to her repertoire.

Carrie was a pioneer in doula education, including social justice and anti-racism content in her trainings when white-led doula institutions overlooked its importance. She introduced hybrid courses that included online content in addition to in-person sessions. She allowed students to attend her classes remotely, opening access to doulas in areas where live trainings weren't available. Finally, Carrie shattered the belief that doula training had to be in-person by launching her fully online course in 2016, long before the COVID-19 pandemic forced everyone online.

Over the years, Carrie has studied with dozens of teachers, mentors, coaches, and trainers to hone her business, marketing, writing, and coaching skills. She weaves psychology, attachment theory, spirituality, and the sacred feminine into all her work. Her goal has always been to not only improve her own knowledge and performance, but to share what she learns with her students.

Carrie has helped hundreds of families welcome their babies into the world, witnessed the remarkable transformation of new parents, and honored the fascinating and powerful process of birth. She has trained thousands of doulas and helped hundreds of them to launch their businesses. She can confidently say she has realized her dream of providing exquisite care to others.

Carrie believes fiercely that doulas are the key to transforming the future of how we care for one another in any of life's challenging situations.

About the Author

Doulas: Changing the world one client at a time.

To contact Carrie for speaking engagements, bulk orders, media inquiries, or just to say "Hi!" visit www.carriekenner.com.

MORE FROM THE AUTHOR

Other titles by Carrie Kenner:

The Becoming a Doula Journal

The Doula Success Formula

Coming Soon

Becoming a Birth Doula (coming Spring 2025)

The Doula Business Workbook

Placenta Encapsulation: The Ultimate Training Manual

Courses & Workshops

Learn more about my courses, business coaching, writing programs, and more at www.carriekenner.com or www.doula-training.carriekenner.com.

Be the first to hear about discounts, new courses, and what I'm offering next. Join my mailing list at www.doula-training.carriekenner.com/contact.

Resources

Join my online community and access more resources at www.doula-training.carriekenner.com/resources.

www.ingramcontent.com/pod-product-compliance
Lightning Source LLC
Chambersburg PA
CBHW080518030426
42337CB00023B/4557